INSTRUCTOR'S MANUAL FOR Clinical Pharmacology and Nursing Management

ROBERTA TODD SPENCER, R.N., M.S.
Adjunct Assistant Professor, College of Nursing
University of Florida, Gainesville, Florida
Associate Professor Emeritus
State University College, Plattsburgh, New York

LYNN WEMETT NICHOLS, B.S.N., M.S.N.
Associate Professor, Department of Nursing
State University of New York, Plattsburgh, New York

GLADYS B. LIPKIN, R.N.C., C.S., M.S., F.A.A.N.
Nurse Psychotherapist in private practice
Childbirth (Lamaze) Instructor; Lecturer
Certified by ANA as Generalist and Specialist
in Psychiatric-Mental Health Nursing and
by ANA and MAACOG in Obstetric Nursing
Bayside, New York

HELEN M. SABO, B.S.N., M.S.N.
Associate Professor, Department of Nursing
State University of New York, Plattsburgh, New York

FRANCES M. WEST, R.N., B.S.N., M.S.N
Vice-President, Nursing Service Division
Champlain Valley Physicians Hospital Medical Center
Plattsburgh, New York

Contributors

Mary X. Britten, R.N., Ed.D.
Associate Professor of Nursing and Coordinator, Graduate Program
State University of New York
Binghamton, New York

Martha Fortune, R.N., M.S.
Holistic Nurse Practitioner
Rochester, New York

Patricia Hryzak Lind, R.N., M.S.
Pediatric Manager, Anthony L. Jordan Health Center
Rochester, New York
Adjunct Faculty, School of Nursing
University of Rochester
Rochester, New York

Charlotte Torres, R.N., M.S
Assistant Professor of Clinical Nursing
School of Nursing
University of Rochester
Rochester, New York

INSTRUCTOR'S MANUAL FOR Clinical Pharmacology and Nursing Management

THIRD EDITION

J. B. LIPPINCOTT COMPANY
Philadelphia
Cambridge New York St. Louis San Francisco
London Singapore Sydney Tokyo

Coordinating Editorial Assistant: Ellen Campbell
Manuscript Editor: Irene Glynn
Production: Till & Till, Inc.
Compositor: C. L. Hutson Company, Inc.
Printer/Binder: Malloy Lithographing, Inc.

Third Edition

6 5 4 3 2 1

ISBN 0-397-54705-6

The author and publisher have exerted every effort to ensure that drug selection and dosage set forth in this text are in accord with current recommendations and practice at the time of publication. However, in view of ongoing research, changes in government regulations, and the constant flow of information relating to drug therapy and drug reactions, the reader is urged to check the package insert for each drug for any change in indications and dosage and for added warnings and precautions. This is particularly important if the recommended agent is a new or infrequently employed drug.

Introduction

The authors and contributors of *Clinical Pharmacology and Nursing Management* have developed this manual to aid instructors and to facilitate student learning. The manual follows the book chapter by chapter, but it is not meant to be a series of complete lesson plans. Rather, it presents examples and gives suggestions that serve as a stimulus for instructors. A variety of ideas are given, but it is our hope that instructors will be motivated to devise some plans unique to their situations. We also welcome your sharing these ideas with us for future editions. But, beyond stimulating instructors in planning for their classes, we also intend to assist instructors in intensifying their students' interests.

Schools vary in the amount of classroom time. Therefore, the material in the textbook and manual may be expanded or reduced to meet the needs of the individual class or the subject matter to be discussed. For instance, Chapter 22 on Autonomic Drugs and Chapter 32 on Steroid Hormones may require more than one class period for adequate coverage of the various drug families.

On the other hand, some of the earlier chapters or later chapters in the book could be combined. An example of a good combination is Chapters 52 and 54 because they discuss community health nursing and over-the-counter drugs.

The Text as a Teaching Tool

The textbook abounds with pedagogic materials. Summaries throughout chapters review main facts. Boxed material highlights other important points. Figures illustrate various aspects of the content. Some line drawings review important details in picture form, other figures illustrate drug administration techniques, and still others pertain to physiology. Tables are provided for reference or review. Bibliographies provide further reading for the student or instructor. The glossary may be used in a variety of ways, and nursing information is easy to find in the chapter outlines on each chapter-opening page and within the text in color. Most of the nursing content is presented in the nursing process format. Illustrative examples of individualized care plans are included.

Each chapter in the text has several Learning and Enrichment Experiences. These are activities that may be adapted to class needs. Learning Experiences include experiences likely to be required of all students, for example, the integration of pharmacological principles in the care of clients in the clinical laboratory. Enrichment Experiences are planned to pique the student's curiosity and to prompt complementary study and experiential activities, beyond the basic, essential curriculum content.

Using the Instructor's Manual

Just as students will find the textbook easy to use, instructors will find the Instructor's Manual an asset to their course planning. Each chapter is divided into four parts: outline, introduction, Teaching Strategies, and Evaluation Examples (Test Items). Chapters begin with a brief outline of the textual material. Not all levels of subheads are given here because of space, but the outlines indicate the basic material. Introductory material delineates the learning focus of the chapter and traces the important concepts to be learned. A section called Teaching Strategies suggests methods of presentation, classroom exercises, field trips, audiovisual aids, guest speakers, or other ideas as tools for the instructor. Activities suggested to reinforce the course material have, in most cases, been performed successfully by the contributors to this book in their own teaching experiences. Teaching Strategies presented in this manual do not include the Learning Experiences that were given in the textbook. The material in this manual gives ideas for additional supplementary work. At the end of each chapter there is a section called Evaluation Examples (Test Items). Methods of evaluation, such as essay questions, multiple choice items, short answer questions, and practical demonstration, are presented briefly.

Other Instructional Materials

The field of pharmacology changes rapidly. It is advantageous to supplement the text with journal articles or to have samples of journals on display so that students may familiarize themselves with ongoing sources of information on pharmacology and drug administration. The school and public libraries may be helpful sources for students. Additional materials are available free or for a minimal charge from various sources. Local representatives of national agencies and other health agencies may give or loan some of their educational materials for classroom or student use, such as brochures and films. Speakers are available from some of these agencies (e.g., the American Heart Association, the American Lung Association, and the American Red Cross). Pharmaceutical companies and your local pharmaceutical representative are other sources of free films. These films are excellent, although their product is mentioned, and students should be made aware of the marketing impact of these films.

Computers have opened a new source for information and experimentation. Information about drugs may be available through computer services in school libraries, medical centers, and the larger health-care institutions.

Exploring for the Future

Students should be encouraged to maximize their knowledge and skills by taking advantage of every learning opportunity available. In the future, these nursing students will contribute to health maintenance and prevention of illness with their knowledge and understanding. However, it is the instructor who makes the material lively and interesting so that the students can enthusiastically explore the field of nursing management in pharmacology.

Contents

UNIT ONE: INTRODUCTION TO PHARMACOLOGY

UNIT TWO: THERAPY WITH DRUGS

UNIT THREE: ADMINISTRATION OF MEDICATIONS

UNIT FOUR: DRUGS USED FOR INFLAMMATIONS AND INFECTIONS

UNIT FIVE: DRUGS AFFECTING THE NERVOUS SYSTEM

UNIT SIX: DRUGS AFFECTING THE CARDIOVASCULAR SYSTEM

UNIT SEVEN: DRUGS AFFECTING THE GASTROINTESTINAL SYSTEM

UNIT EIGHT: DRUGS AFFECTING THE ENDOCRINE SYSTEM

UNIT NINE: DRUGS AFFECTING SPECIFIC BODY SYSTEMS

UNIT TEN: DRUGS USED FOR NEOPLASTIC DISEASE

UNIT ELEVEN: DRUGS AFFECTING THE IMMUNE SYSTEM

UNIT TWELVE: NUTRITIONAL SUPPLEMENTS

UNIT THIRTEEN: MISCELLANEOUS DRUG FAMILIES

UNIT FOURTEEN: SPECIAL CONSIDERATIONS IN DRUG THERAPY

UNIT ONE: INTRODUCTION TO PHARMACOLOGY

1
Orientation to Pharmacology: Historical Overview

Scope of Pharmacology
An Interdisciplinary Study
History of Pharmacology
Prehistoric/Primitive Era
Ancient Civilizations
Medieval to Modern Times
Modern Medicine
The Future—A Balance
Nursing Implications
Significance of Pharmacology in Nursing
Pharmacology in Nursing Education

Chapter 1 defines pharmacology in broad terms, presents an abbreviated history of the discipline, and delineates its relationship to the practice of nursing. This material can be used to help the student understand and appreciate the complexity of the subject, the potential of drug use for therapeutic and abusive purposes, and the importance of pharmacology in nursing care.

The study of pharmacology involves the application of principles from both the physical (*i.e.*, material) and social sciences. The student must apply knowledge of such disciplines as chemistry, physiology, psychology, and anthropology to understand the effects of drugs on people. If a course in pharmacology precedes or coincides with the beginning of nursing courses in the curriculum, it may provide the student with a prototype for the application of basic knowledge to the health field, an important scholarly skill in professional nursing.

The history of pharmacology implies that the use of chemicals can confer an adaptive advantage on groups of people. These beneficial effects derive from the successful treatment of disease, the fostering of social unification (*e.g.*, hallucinogens used in religious rites of American Indian tribes), and, in some cases, the exercise of social control (*e.g.*, the use of tranquilizers to control the behavior of persons identified as dissident or mentally ill). Drug use also poses risks. Inappropriate dosing (*e.g.*, purging in appendicitis) can kill the sick person. Indiscriminate use of psychotropic substances can sap the functional effectiveness of individual persons and, if widespread, of groups of people. The use of drugs in every society has been accompanied by some system of legal or moral control. This seems to be necessary to optimal use of chemicals.

The place of pharmacology in nursing is described in relation to the prevention of health problems, early detection of health problems, acute care of the ill, and convalescence. Pharmacology is relevant to nursing at every stage.

Through study of this chapter, the student can be assisted to develop the following concepts:

1 □ The study of pharmacology is complex and multidisciplinary and involves the application of principles from basic physical and social sciences.
2 □ Current trends in the use of chemicals arise from historical developments in pharmacology.
3 □ The use of chemicals involves potential for both benefits and risks.
4 □ Knowledge, judgment, and control are required for optimal use of drugs.
5 □ Pharmacology is highly pertinent to health disciplines including nursing; knowledge and skills related to this discipline are needed at all levels of nursing.

Teaching Strategies

1 □ Classroom discussion may be stimulated by consideration of questions such as the following:
- **a.** What adaptive advantages are conferred on societies using drug substances? (Improved health care, increased social cohesiveness, and social control)
- **b.** What risks attend the use of chemicals? (Toxic or harmful reactions, impaired function, injustice)
- **c.** What factors promote optimal use of drugs? (Knowledge, skill, judgment, and control)

2 □ Plan a debate for class. Resolved: the use of chemicals as drugs is dangerous and should be kept to an absolute minimum. (The arguments presented are likely to represent polar attitudes. Exposing the fallacies of both pro and con positions illustrates the need for avoidance of extreme bias.)

3 □ Ask students to complete Learning Experience 1–1 and bring their self-evaluations to class. To demonstrate the range of attitudes, have students write down their "permissiveness-avoidance score." Preserving anonymity, arrange the data in a frequency distribution that reveals a class profile. Class discussion might consider the following:
- **a.** What kinds of factors (*e.g.*, historical trends, cultural practices, family tradition, personal experiences) influenced the development of attitudes and values related to drug use?
- **b.** What effect could attitudes and values have on nursing judgment in matters relating to the administration of drugs or the care of chemically dependent clients?

Instructors who have analyzed their own attitudes toward drugs, acknowledged their own biases, and taken measures to compensate for their influence on nursing judgment might share this experience with students.

Evaluation Examples (Test Items)

ESSAY QUESTIONS

1. Briefly trace the history of the use of one psychotropic drug (alcohol, opium, or marijuana) to the present time. In view of this history, do you think the use of the substance should be legal in the United States? Explain why or why not.

2. Describe the relationship between pharmacology and the basic sciences: chemistry, biology, sociology, and psychology.

*MULTIPLE CHOICE ITEMS**

1. According to the text Clinical Pharmacology and Nursing Management, pharmacology is best defined as the study of
- *1. Chemical effects on living tissues
- 2. Medicinal drugs
- 3. Chemicals with toxic properties
- 4. Chemical pollution

2. The study of pharmacology may require application of knowledge from the following sciences:
- a. Chemistry
- b. Biology
- c. Geology
- d. Sociology
- e. Psychology
- 1. a, b
- 2. a, b, c
- 3. a, b, d, e
- 4. d, e
- *5. All of the above

3. When did the study of pharmacology begin?
- *1. In prehistoric times, through trial and error
- 2. About 3000 years BC in China
- 3. About 2000 years BC in Egypt
- 4. During the Renaissance, when chemical research began

4. The earliest known written record of drug use was found in
- 1. Egypt
- 2. Sumer
- *3. China
- 4. Greece

5. Coca (cocaine) was first used by natives of
- 1. Northern Africa
- 2. Southeast Asia
- *3. Central and South America
- 4. Europe and western Asia

6. Homeopathic medicine involves the use of
- 1. Purging and bloodletting
- *2. Drug preparations in highly diluted forms
- 3. Drug preparations in relatively concentrated forms
- 4. Natural medicine

7. In modern nursing practice, the nurse is expected to
- a. Administer drugs accurately, in strict accord with the physician's orders
- b. Teach clients how to use drug substances for optimal effect on health
- c. Assess client responses to drug therapy
- 1. a, b
- *2. b, c
- 3. a, c
- 4. All of the above

*Throughout the Instructor's Manual, the correct answers to multiple choice items are indicated by an asterisk (*).

2 Standards and Controls

Drug Controls
- *International Controls*
- *National Controls*
- *State Controls*
- *Local Regulations*
- *Institutional Controls*
- *Individual Control*
- *Nursing Implications*

Drug Standards
- *Purity*
- *Potency*
- *Bioavailability*
- *Efficacy*
- *Safety/Toxicity*
- *Testing Procedures*
- *Nursing Implications*

Chapter 2 discusses legal, institutional, and informal controls over drug use and the standards established for control of the quality of manufactured drug preparations. Legislative controls in effect in the United States and Canada are discussed in detail. Criteria for evaluating drug preparations are listed and discussed.

Through the study of this chapter, the student may develop the following concepts:

1 □ Formal or informal controls on the use of pharmacologically active substances are imposed by all cultures.

2 □ Formal controls include institutional policies, procedures, and laws providing for the establishment of official pharmacopoeia, standards for the production of drugs, and restrictions on the sale and use of drugs.

3 □ Informal controls include family practices, cultural taboos, mores, and customs.

4 □ The strictness of controls on the use of drugs tends to be inversely related to the size of the social unit imposing them.

5 □ The consent of the client is the final control on use of drugs.

Teaching Strategies

Classroom discussion could focus on regulations governing drug use in the local community as one example of the impact of these regulations on nursing practice. Policies of local health-care agencies should be studied in relation to the following: the formal basis for imposition of the control (federal, state, local, or institutional directive); procedures used for implementing the controls; and required documentation (charts and records). Students should also consider the measures nurses may take to become acquainted with local regulations when beginning nursing practice in a new institution or community.

Evaluation Examples (Test Items)

ESSAY QUESTIONS

1. Compare and contrast state regulations governing the use of narcotics such as morphine in a hospital setting with the policies and procedures of a local hospital. Discuss briefly the rationale underlying the adoption by the hospital of controls that differ from those required by the government.

2. Briefly relate the history of prohibition of the sale of alcoholic beverages in the United States. Discuss the arguments for and against legal prohibitions of drug substances in common use, such as alcohol.

TRUE AND FALSE STATEMENTS

F **1.** Drug experience reports submitted to the Food and Drug Administration (FDA) must originate with a physician or dentist.

F **2.** Drugs classified under Schedule 1 of the Controlled Substance Act of 1970 are medicinal agents with the greatest potential for causing dependence.

T **3.** At present there is no legally sanctioned medicinal use for heroin in the United States.

F **4.** In the United States, prescriptions for narcotics such as morphine may be refilled only once before renewal.

F **5.** According to federal FDA regulations, medicinal drugs sold in the United States must be 100% pure.

SHORT ANSWER QUESTION

Define the following terms relating to drug preparations:

Purity	Bioavailability
Potency	Efficacy

MULTIPLE CHOICE ITEMS

1. The first narcotic control act passed by any nation was
1. The Food, Drug, and Cosmetic Act of 1906
*2. The Harrison Act of 1914
3. The Food, Drug, and Cosmetic Act of 1938
4. The Durham–Humphrey Amendment of 1952

2. Official pharmacopoeiae of the United States include

a. United States Pharmacopoeia and National Formulary
b. British Pharmacopoeia
c. Physicians' Desk Reference

*1. a
2. b
3. c
4. a, c
5. All of the above

3. According to the Durham–Humphrey Amendment of 1952, "legend" drugs are those that

1. Have been used as traditional remedies by folk healers
2. May be sold over the counter without a prescription
*3. Require a prescription from a qualified health professional
4. Require a prescription, which must be renewed every 6 months

4. The area of enforcement undertaken most recently by the Food and Drug Administration is the standard for

1. Purity
2. Potency
3. Bioavailability
*4. Efficacy
5. Safety/toxicity

5. The area of enforcement for which we still lack reliable tests for establishing standards is that of

1. Purity
2. Potency
*3. Bioavailability
4. Efficacy
5. Safety/toxicity

3 Nursing Process in the Management of Drug-Related Problems

Assessment
Data Base
Analysis
Diagnosis
Planning
Intervention
Evaluation
Nursing Process and General Drug Problems

Chapter 3 deals with the application of the nursing process in the treatment of responses to drugs and chemicals, particularly the independent functions of the nurse caring for clients on therapeutic drug regimens. The pharmacologic aspects of each step in the nursing process are outlined, with specific examples of nursing diagnoses, objectives, goals, and criteria for evaluation. A nursing care plan is presented as a model for clinical situations in which the drug regimen is a critical factor in the care of the client.

Through study of this chapter, the student can be assisted to develop the following concepts:

1 □ The nurse caring for clients receiving therapeutic medications carries out many independent as well as dependent functions to enhance the client's response to the drug regimen and to reduce the risk of adverse reactions.
2 □ The logical, scientific, problem-solving approach inherent in the nursing process is applicable to pharmacologic aspects of care.
3 □ Facts about the properties of drugs in use must be included in the data base used for assessment.
4 □ Diagnoses in situations involving drug regimens should include both actual and potential problems arising from the use of medications.
5 □ Nursing diagnoses related to drug regimens may indicate the potential for adverse effects from the drugs, a client's need for teaching, or compliance with the regimen.
6 □ Clients' responses to drug therapy are influenced by many factors, including their knowledge about and attitudes toward drugs, functional capacities, and financial security.
7 □ The nurse works cooperatively with the client, physician, and pharmacist to achieve optimum response to drug therapy.
8 □ Client teaching is an important element in the care of those receiving therapeutic drugs, especially in regard to noninstitutionalized clients who manage their own drug regimens.
9 □ Nursing care plans for clients receiving therapeutic drugs are similar to other care plans in structure; they require an adequate data base, clear objectives and goals, and measurable criteria for evaluation.

Teaching Strategies

If students beginning the study of pharmacology have already been introduced to the nursing process, the study of this chapter should reinforce the material that has been taught previously. The use of the nursing process in the care of clients receiving therapeutic drugs should serve as an example of the application of basic principles, rather than as a departure from the usual practice. If the study of pharmacology precedes the introduction to nursing practice, this chapter may be postponed until laboratory experiences in the clinical setting begin to incorporate the administration of drugs into the student's experience. This chapter is inappropriate for the beginning study of the nursing process and for the development of nursing care plans.

□ Skill in developing nursing care plans requires practice. In relation to the study of this chapter, students should be involved in writing care plans for real (or realistically simulated) clinical situations. Among the drugs that could be used as examples of therapeutic medications are, for short-term therapy, penicillin, DPT vaccine, or barium sulfate and, for long-term therapy, cimetidine, phenytoin, aspirin in an antirheumatic dosage, or hydrochlorothiazide.

Evaluation Example (Test Item)

OPEN BOOK EXAMINATION

Develop a nursing care plan dealing with drug-related needs of the following client:

Ms. AT, age 32 years, has just been diagnosed as having pulmonary tuberculosis involving the apex of the left lung. She is to be treated as an outpatient with daily dosages of both isoniazid and rifampin.

AT lives in a one-family suburban house with her husband and two children, Christine, 8 years old, and Donald, 10 years old. She has been working part-time as a typist for a temporary agency, "mostly to get out of the house," because her husband's income is generally adequate for the family's needs. Her general physical condition is good, despite the spontaneous loss of about 10 pounds over the last 3 months. Her varied interests include jogging 3 miles at least three times a week, working with the local Girl Scout troop, and doing such handicrafts as knitting and quilting. Her husband and children have been tine-tested for sensitivity to the tuberculosis bacterium, with negative results. AT takes no drugs except a daily maintenance vitamin and mineral preparation and an occasional dose of aspirin for minor pain such as headache.

4

Development of a Knowledge Base in Pharmacology

A Personal Drug File
- *Name of Drug*
- *Drug Family*
- *Desired Therapeutic Effects*
- *Side Effects*
- *Adverse Reactions*
- *Toxic Effects*
- *Contraindications*
- *Dosage Range and Administration Route*
- *Elimination*
- *Nursing Implications*

Sources of Drug Information
- *Pharmacopeiae*
- *Textbooks*
- *Journals*
- *Subscription Services*
- *Package Inserts and the PDR*
- *The Pharmacist*
- *Drug Firms*
- *Supplementary Information*

Nursing Implications

Chapter 4 presents an approach to the study of pharmacology that will help the student to develop sound scholarly methods of inquiry into pharmacology and to build a knowledge base in that discipline. Specific suggestions are provided for study techniques. Current sources of drug information are discussed in relation to criteria for evaluating the usefulness of reference works.

Through the study of this chapter, students may develop the following concepts:

1 □ Current information on drugs is too voluminous for mastery by rote memorization.
2 □ Knowledge of the general properties of the various classes of drugs enables practitioners to develop a reliable data base quickly for use in specific clinical situations.
3 □ Memorization of facts about commonly used drugs helps nurses to maintain an adequate work pace during clinical practice.
4 □ Sound scholarship is required for maintaining an adequate background of information about drugs.

Teaching Strategies

Students need to become familiar with various resources for gathering drug data. This can be encouraged through library assignments, group projects, or classroom activities requiring practice in the use of various drug data sources. Resources may include those found in nursing-care units, institutional pharmacies, and the libraries of schools or health-care agencies. Instructors may wish to share their personal library during a class session. Pharmacists often have useful resources that they allow students to use.

Students beginning clinical practice often find it helpful to make data summaries of each medication prescribed for their clients. If the instructor reads and evaluates these summaries, students may be guided in refining their scholarly skills. This practice provides the foundation for safe habits in administering drugs. If drug summaries are required through the period of clinical practice during which students begin to administer drug doses, the habit of gathering drug data will be well established. Students will then be unlikely to attempt to administer drugs without having adequate information about the prescribed preparations.

Evaluation Examples (Test Items)

ESSAY QUESTIONS

1. List and briefly describe the types of information needed about a drug preparation to give safe care to the client receiving it.

2. Discuss the various meanings of the term "drug sensitivity."

SHORT ANSWER QUESTION

Define the following terms relating to drugs:

Mechanisms of action	Adverse reactions
Therapeutic effects	Side effects
Therapeutic uses	Toxic effects
Indications for prescription	Idiosyncratic reactions
Contraindications	Allergic reactions

MATCHING QUESTION

For the following questions, mark the number(s) on the answer sheet corresponding to the appropriate choice(s):

1. Physicians' Desk Reference
2. United States Pharmacopoeia and National Formulary
3. Drug Information

1. Lists drugs screened for safety and therapeutic effects by a group of experts commissioned by the federal government *(2)*

2. Is most apt to offer information regarding very new brand name drugs *(1)*

3. Is produced by the Hospital Pharmaceutical Association *(3)*

4. Is revised yearly *(1 and 3)*

MULTIPLE CHOICE ITEM

1. When information about a drug is difficult to obtain from printed sources, the nurse is most likely to receive the needed information promptly and reliably from

1. A nursing supervisor
2. A physician
*3. A pharmacist
4. The drug company that produces the medication

5
Toxicology

Access Routes of Toxic Substances
- *Percutaneous Route*
- *Gastrointestinal Route*
- *Parenteral Route*
- *Inhalation Route*

Scope of Poisoning
- *Causes of Poisoning*

Poison Management
- *Information*
- *First Aid for Acute Poisoning or Exposure*
- *Administering an Antidote*
- *Eliminating the Poison*
- *Poison Prevention*

Lead Poisoning
- *Pathophysiology*
- *Signs and Symptoms*
- *Intervention*
- *Prevention*

Mercury Poisoning
- *Pathophysiology*
- *Signs and Symptoms*
- *Interventions*

Toxins in the Hospital Environment
- *Surgical Hazards*
- *Chemical Sterilants*
- *Chemical Disinfectants*

Chemotherapy

Nursing Management

Chapter 5 provides the student with basic knowledge about the science of toxicology. The information presented is intended to familiarize the student with the nature of toxic substances and the routes of exposure most commonly experienced by humans. In addition, statistics about the occurrence of accidental poisoning are cited to draw attention to the community health aspects of poison control and education.

Management of an acute poisoning episode is discussed in detail with guidelines for first aid and emergency room treatment stipulated. Resources for up-to-date information on product contents are identified. Chronic poisoning with heavy metals is also explored. Current preferences in the treatment of lead poisoning are outlined. Educational options for health promotion are included in the discussion of nursing implications.

Through the study of this chapter, the student may develop the following concepts:

1 □ The science of toxicology is multidimensional and includes the study of the effects of chemical substances on biologic systems.

2 □ Exposure to toxic substances produces various responses in different people. The response depends on the nature of the substance, the dose, the susceptibility of the person, biologic factors, and the route of entry.

3 □ Children under the age of 5 years are at high risk for accidental poisoning.

4 □ When involved in a poison emergency, treat the person first, then the poison.

5 □ The goal of poison management is to remove or eliminate the poison.

6 □ Poisoning accidents are preventable through consumer awareness and education.

7 □ Children between the ages of 12 and 36 months are at risk for plumbism.

8 □ Absorption of lead into the body may affect multiple body systems.

Teaching Strategies

1 □ Classroom discussion of the nurse's role in poison prevention and treatment may be influenced by the presence or absence of a community health experience at the time of study.

2 □ Assignment of the learning experiences may facilitate firsthand observation of selected poison prevention programs, depending on availability of such programs within the community.

3 □ Library research will facilitate acquisition of current statistics from such programs within the community.

4 □ A presentation by local public health officials would be useful to provide information regarding the presence of toxic hazards within a given community. Governmental regulations to prevent contamination and protect the environment could also be explored in this forum.

Evaluation Examples (Test Items)

ESSAY AND SHORT ANSWER QUESTIONS

1. Define and differentiate among environmental, economic, and forensic toxicology.

2. Identify four access routes for poisons in the human body and give one example of a poison per route.

3. Identify the seven steps for first aid in a poisoning emergency.

4. List ten principles for prevention of household poisoning.

MULTIPLE CHOICE ITEMS

1. According to the National Clearinghouse for Poison Control Centers, the most frequent cause of death by ingestion in children under the age of 5 years is

1. Ingestion of cosmetics
*2. Ingestion of analgesics
3. Ingestion of plants
4. Ingestion of antipyretics

2. Which of the following is *not* a contraindication for inducing emesis in a poison victim?

1. Absence of gag reflex
*2. Ingestion of aspirin
3. Ingestion of corrosives
4. Ingestion of volatile hydrocarbons

3. Which of the following would most strongly support a positive diagnosis of plumbism?

1. Presence of behavioral symptoms
2. Presence of abdominal pain and vomiting
3. History of pica
*4. Two successive venous blood lead levels of ≥ 70 µg/dl

UNIT TWO: THERAPY WITH DRUGS

6

Approaches to Drug Therapy

Three Major Approaches
Magical Approach
Empirical Approach
Rational Approach
Nursing Management
Nursing Implications
Client Education

Chapter 6 describes the evolution of pharmacology and presents a brief overview of the magical, empiric, and rational approaches to the development and use of chemical substances for therapeutic purposes. The material presented will assist the student to recognize the relationship among folk practices and beliefs, knowledge about cause and effect, and scientific methodologies for problem solving. The ability to make use of medicines and the development of basic health practice emerged from these relationships.

By studying this chapter, the student should develop the following concepts:

1 □ The development of medicine parallels advancements made in the use of scientific methodologies.
2 □ Modern pharmacology evolved from oral tribal traditions, cultural traditions of environmental uses, and chemical and biologic methodologies.
3 □ The magical approach resulted from superstition and fear because there was little knowledge of the cause-and-effect relationship of disease and illness in ancient civilizations.
4 □ The empiric approach relates drug use to experience.
5 □ The rational approach developed at the end of the 18th century when problem-solving methods began to be used in the evaluation of drugs.
6 □ Modern health-care practice continues to reflect the magical, empiric, and rational orientations.
7 □ Nurses, in certain roles, are in advantageous positions to educate clients and to promote a wellness orientation.

Teaching Strategies

1 □ Use classroom discussion to explore the following questions:
- **a.** What folk practices in the use of home remedies are carried out in one's family? Which approach(es) to modern pharmacology do they represent?
- **b.** What expectations do consumers have about the purpose of medicines when seeking health care?

2 □ Present the following case for discussion:

A 24-year-old man sought medical treatment for a severe sore throat and symptoms of a common cold presenting as upper respiratory congestion, fever, and productive cough. The onset of symptoms was 5 days earlier. He related that he had been using hot honey-and-lemon tea and gargling with warm salt water for his throat. He had also used some antibiotics that a friend had given him but he had not experienced any relief of symptoms. Aspirin was being used to reduce the fever. The physician examined the patient, took a throat culture, and prescribed another antibiotic, with instructions for the patient to call back for test results in 2 days.
- **a.** Discuss the nature of the health care sought, identifying the types of approaches used in the initial efforts at self-care.
- **b.** Discuss the nature of the health care delivered, identifying the rationale for the approach taken.
- **c.** Discuss the probable expectations this consumer had in seeking medical advice.

Evaluation Examples (Test Items)

ESSAY QUESTIONS

1. Trace the evolution of modern pharmacology, identifying the three major areas of development.

2. Discuss the development of the rational approach to pharmacology, identifying five areas of scientific exploration essential to the study of medicines.

7 Pharmacodynamics and Pharmacokinetics

Pharmacodynamics
- *Alteration of Cellular Environments*
- *Provision of Substrate Material*
- *Alteration of the Speed of Cell Functions*
- *Nursing Implications*

Pharmacokinetics
- *Drug Absorption*
- *Drug Distribution*
- *Drug Biotransformation*
- *Drug Excretion*
- *Interaction of Pharmacokinetic Processes*
- *Nursing Implications*

Chapter 7 describes the mechanisms by which drugs move through the body and exert their physiologic effects. Mechanisms at the cellular and molecular levels are stressed. Included in the discussion are the cell receptor theory of drug action, processes of membrane transport, physiologic and environmental factors influencing the distribution of drugs, and routes of absorption, distribution, metabolism and excretion. The blood-brain barrier, the movement of drugs across the placenta, and the secretion of drugs in milk are also described.

Through a study of this chapter, students may develop the following concepts:

1 □ The actions of drugs involve cellular or molecular processes that can explain their physiologic effects.
2 □ The laws of chemistry and physics apply to the processes of pharmacodynamics.
3 □ Drugs act by various mechanisms to exert their physiologic effects.
4 □ A single drug may act by several mechanisms and may exert multiple effects.
5 □ Some drugs (agonists) interact with special receptors on cell membranes; others (antagonists) inhibit these interactions.
6 □ Drugs may act locally, in the area of the body in which they are applied, or systemically, at a site or sites distant from the area of application; systemic effects require wide distribution of the drug by the circulating blood.
7 □ Movement of drugs in the body conforms to the physical and chemical laws affecting the kinetics of matter.
8 □ Drugs may be stored in tissue depots; stored drugs generally exert few physiologic effects.
9 □ Drug concentration decreases exponentially with the passage of time; the serum half-life of a drug is equal to the time required for a 50% reduction in serum concentration. After seven serum half-lives have elapsed, serum concentration is less than 1% of the original concentration, and drug action is considered to have ceased.

Teaching Strategies

The content of this chapter is largely theoretic. The processes discussed in the text are difficult to demonstrate in any real sense, but audiovisual materials may demonstrate them symbolically.

1 □ The use of pertinent clinical material as examples of practical consequences of these processes can help students to apply the theory of nursing practice. Clinical illustrations of the significance of pharmacodynamic and pharmacokinetic theory might include examples such as the following:
- **a.** A comparison of drug regimens involving rapid-acting preparations and depot preparations of the same drug (*e.g.*, crystalline penicillin and procaine penicillin in a waxy base when administered by injection, regular and long-lasting insulins)
- **b.** A comparison of the time required for alleviation of pain by oral and intramuscular administration of drugs such as meperidine
- **c.** The necessity for administration of drugs by injection because they are ineffective when given orally (*e.g.*, insulin)
- **d.** Drug regimens for clients receiving periodic hemodialysis

2 □ Although many examples are cited in the text, it is more effective to elicit examples from the students. The materials may thereby be related to students' experiences. If students are involved in clinical laboratory, illustrative examples may be drawn from these experiences.
3 □ As much as possible, class time should be devoted to discussion rather than lecture. Ample time should be allowed for questions.
4 □ As a classroom exercise, students may be asked to compute the number of serum half-lives that must elapse before serum concentration from a single dose falls below 1% of maximum concentration.

Evaluation Examples (Test Items)

ESSAY QUESTIONS

1. Describe the mechanisms of action of opioid drugs and opioid (narcotic) antagonists, giving examples of each class of drugs.

2. Trace the movement through the tissues of a drug administered intramuscularly, identifying the pharmacokinetic processes involved. Assume that the drug is a protein-bound acidic salt that does not cross the blood–brain barrier and is excreted as a glucuronide.

SHORT ANSWER QUESTION

Define the following terms as related to drugs:

Agonist	Active transport
Antagonist	Enteric coating
Cell receptor	Enterohepatic cycle
Pinocytosis	Serum half-life

MULTIPLE CHOICE ITEMS

1. The most important organ for drug excretion is
1. The liver
2. The intestine
3. The skin
*4. The kidney

2. Biotransformation of drugs occurs mainly in the microsomal portion of liver cells. The purposes of biotransformation are to
a. Facilitate excretion
b. Facilitate detoxification
c. Delay elimination
d. Prolong absorption time
*1. a, b
2. a, d
3. b, c
4. b, d
5. All of these

3. Rapid loss of weight is most likely to precipitate spontaneous poisoning by the pollutant
1. Sulfur dioxide
*2. DDT
3. Plutonium
4. Lead

4. In an adult with normally functioning liver and kidneys, the time interval required for most drugs to clear the body (and to ensure that interactions with other drugs will not occur) is
1. 24 hours
2. 48 hours
3. 1 week
*4. 2 weeks

5. Microsomal enzymes involved in drug metabolism are susceptible to the action of drugs. Enzyme stimulation will
a. Accelerate excretion
b. Facilitate deactivation
c. Increase toxicity of the drug
d. Accelerate activation of most drugs
*1. a, b
2. a, d
3. b, c
4. b, d
5. All of these

6. An example of an enzyme stimulator is
1. Maalox
2. Atropine
3. Hexobarbital
*4. Phenobarbital

7. Why is epinephrine mixed with local anesthetics such as procaine before they are injected?
1. To increase effectiveness of the drugs by addition
2. To prevent systemic toxic effects by antagonizing the side effect of the anesthetic
3. To slow absorption into the systemic circulation by producing a relatively insoluble complex
*4. To slow absorption into the systemic circulation by local vasoconstriction

8. What type of chemicals are most likely to be absorbed by the skin?
1. Highly saturated fatty acids
*2. Volatile hydrocarbons
3. Carbohydrates
4. Inorganic salts

8
Drug Preparations

Drug Nomenclature
Chemical Name
Generic Name
Official Name
Trade Name
Abbreviations
Drug Families
Nursing Management
Sources of Drugs
Plant Kingdom
Animal Kingdom
Mineral Resources
Synthetic Chemicals
Nursing Management
Drug Constituents
Active Ingredients
Additives
Nursing Management
Types of Preparations
Solid Forms
Semi-solid Medications
Liquids
Nursing Management

Chapter 8 focuses on basic knowledge of drug preparations. The student is introduced to the classification of drugs according to chemical structure, generic name, official name, trade name, and drug family. Drugs prepared from sources in the plant and animal kingdoms, mineral resources, and synthetic processes are described to demonstrate the wealth of drug resources. This chapter describes both active ingredients and the various additives used in drug formulations. Common types of preparations are defined.

Implications of unsafe drug practices are discussed in the nursing process sections. The professional nurse's role as client educator is explored. A sound theoretic foundation of drug therapy is emphasized to ensure intelligent and safe administration of medicinal drugs.

Through the study of this chapter, students may develop the following concepts:

1 □ A basic understanding of drug classification systems is necessary to intelligent and safe use of all drugs.
2 □ Drugs are classified according to their chemical structures, generic names, official names, trade names, and drug families.
3 □ Therapeutic effects of drugs are influenced by the dosage and type of drug preparation.
4 □ The safe and effective practice of drug administration requires knowledge of the drug's active ingredients and other constituents.
5 □ When a drug's name is capitalized, it is probably a trade name; chemical, generic, and official names are written without capitalization.
6 □ A specific drug has one official and one generic name, but may have numerous trade names.
7 □ Acronym abbreviations should not be used unless they have been adopted formally and listed in written procedures or policies.
8 □ A single drug may be classified as a member of a number of drug families; a family name may denote chemical structure, mode of action, physiologic action, or therapeutic effect.
9 □ Familiarity with alternative names of drugs is required for accurate identification of medicines taken by a client.
10 □ A complete drug history is the basis for analysis of and counseling about the drug regimen.
11 □ Nurses collaborate with clients, physicians, and pharmacists to develop optimal drug regimens.
12 □ Inaccurate transcription of drug orders may result in an error in medication.
13 □ Drugs are produced from plant, animal, and mineral sources and from synthetic processes (including recombinant DNA techniques.)
14 □ A complete drug history includes information about client allergies as well as a list of all medicinal substances used.
15 □ Trade name preparations of a given drug may produce different responses in a client because of variations in salt form or additives used.
16 □ When drugs are manufactured in forms that resemble candy in appearance and taste, the risk of poisoning due to accidental ingestion, especially by children, is increased.
17 □ Drug formulations are usually designed for administration by a single route; substitution for administration by another route can be dangerous, ineffective, or both.
18 □ Nurses must be able to recognize the potential for harm of an inappropriate drug order.
19 □ Nurses should be able to suggest acceptable alternative drugs for a client's regimen.

Teaching Strategies

1 □ Selected activities may be assigned to elicit discussion by small groups of four to six students:

a. Identify the "cold remedy" product(s) you would purchase for your sick child (2 years old) and your grandparent (80 years old). Were the products different for each? Why or why not? Were you aware of all the ingredients contained in those cold remedies?

b. Discuss the professional, ethical, and legal dilemmas nurses may encounter when refusing to follow an incompletely or illegibly written medication order on a client's hospital or nursing home chart. A problem, preferably taken from actual clinical experience, might be presented in the first person on a tape or cassette.

2 □ Plan a tour of a pharmaceutical company. Before the tour, remind students that some presentations will be slanted. Follow the tour by discussion to disclose biased viewpoints.

3 □ Arrange a display of all kinds of preparations. Ask students to identify them and relate the rationale behind their use.

Evaluation Examples (Test Items)

TRUE AND FALSE STATEMENTS

_F_ **1.** The generic name of a drug is usually the same as its chemical name.

_F_ **2.** In the United States, official names are printed in Drug Information, published by the United States Pharmacopoeia Association.

_T_ **3.** A drug may have many proprietary names.

_F_ **4.** The United States Pharmacopoeia and National Formulary publishes a list of approved acronym abbreviations for drug names.

_F_ **5.** Nurses should not reveal to the client the names of prescribed drugs unless the physician has asked that the name be listed on the prescription label.

_T_ **6.** Enteric-coated tablets are designed to delay the release of their ingredients until they reach the intestinal mucosa.

SHORT ANSWER QUESTION

Define and give an example of each of the following terms:

Generic name	Vehicles
Official name	Fillers
Active ingredient	Diluents
Additive	Binders
Alkaloid	Disintegrators
Glycosides	Lubricants
Polypeptides	Flavorings
Steroids	Dyes

MULTIPLE CHOICE ITEMS

1. If a drug name is capitalized, it is most likely to be a

1. Chemical name
2. Generic name
3. Official name

*4. Trade name

2. A concise, distinctive drug name that has been adopted by the United States Adopted Name Council would most likely be the

1. Chemical name

*2. Generic name

3. Official name
4. Brand name

3. The source of aspirin is

1. The plant kingdom
2. The animal kingdom

*3. Mineral resources

4. Laboratory synthesis

4. Recombinant DNA techniques are utilized in the manufacture of drugs derived from

1. The plant kingdom
2. The animal kingdom
3. Mineral resources

*4. Laboratory synthesis

5. The drug potassium chloride would be classified as a(n)

*1. Salt

2. Steroid
3. Alkaloid
4. Polypeptide

6. Drugs most likely to act as ions (electrically charged particles) are

*1. Salts

2. Steroids
3. Alkaloids
4. Polypeptides

7. An example of a glycoside is

1. Insulin
2. Morphine sulfate

*3. Digitalis

4. Testosterone

9 Drug Reactions and Interactions

Chapter 9 discusses adverse reactions and the principles behind drug interactions. Every physiologically active drug has the potential to cause an undesirable reaction that may induce illness. Adverse reactions are of many types and include side effects, allergic reactions, idiosyncratic reactions, chain reactions, cumulative reactions, and tolerance and dependence.

Drug interactions are varied and may affect the absorption, distribution, biotransformation, or excretion of drugs. They may be beneficial or hazardous and may differ from person to person. They may be of major clinical significance or of no clinical significance at all.

As the health-care practitioner with the closest and most prolonged contact with the client, the nurse bears a heavy responsibility for protecting the client from adverse reactions and interactions. This chapter emphasizes that the best way for the nurse to be prepared is to understand the basic mechanisms of reactions and interactions instead of depending on reference to lists of reported reactions and interactions. This chapter also describes the nursing care for common drug-related problems.

Through study of this chapter, students may develop the following concepts:

1 □ Because they change or influence body function, all effective drugs have a potential for toxicity.
2 □ The likelihood of a drug causing toxicity is inversely related to that drug's safety margin.
3 □ Adverse reactions to drugs vary in the body tissues affected, in their severity, and in the time required for onset of symptoms.
4 □ Identification of adverse reactions to new drugs requires several years of clinical experience in the medical use of the drug.
5 □ Iatrogenic conditions arising from drug use may take the form of toxic states, allergic reactions, disease syndromes similar to diseases occurring in the absence of drug use, and withdrawal syndromes that occur when drugs are discontinued.
6 □ The likelihood of iatrogenic illness increases as the number of drugs used concurrently increases.
7 □ Drug cumulation occurs whenever the rate of absorption exceeds the rate of metabolism and excretion.
8 □ Toxic states usually become evident when drug concentrations in the body reach a certain critical level.
9 □ Toxic states caused by cumulation are most likely to occur when drugs that have a narrow safety margin are taken for a prolonged period of time.
10 □ Interactions during absorption result in an increase or decrease in the relative rate of absorption, or an increase or decrease in the amount of drug that is absorbed, or both.
11 □ Interactions during absorption may result from direct interaction of the drugs, insufficient ingestion of a solvent, or dissolution rate changes.
12 □ Many drugs are bound to plasma proteins; the bound fraction has no pharmacologic activity and the therapeutically important concentration is that of the free, unbound drug.
13 □ Drugs do compete with other drugs for drug-binding sites and can displace bound drugs, but the importance of *in vivo* protein-binding-displacement interactions has probably been exaggerated. After displacement there is a transient increase in free drug concentration, but the drug's rate of clearance is also usually increased, which decreases the significance of the displacement.
14 □ Many drugs can displace natural body chemicals from their storage locations in various depots in the body. The displaced chemicals may contribute to the drug's effect(s).
15 □ A drug may inhibit the metabolism of another drug or an endogenous compound such as an enzyme with desirable or undesirable effects.
16 □ Drugs may increase the synthesis of drug-metabolizing enzymes, affecting the intensity and duration of action of many drugs.
17 □ Two drugs may compete for tubular transport, with the result that the tubular secretion of one of them is decreased.
18 □ Alkalinization of urine increases the rate of excretion of acidic drugs, whereas acidification of urine increases the urinary excretion rate of basic drugs.

Teaching Strategies

Students encountering clients who experience adverse reactions to a drug or drug interactions should be referred to this chapter for a background of knowledge for the study of the specific problem under consideration. This chapter will also be useful for students who have difficulty understanding the types of adverse ions,

rug interactions discussed in the chap- k describing drug families. If an intro- se in pharmacology precedes or accompa- nical courses in the nursing curriculum, ion of this chapter would be appropriate cology is studied. The content of this chapter self to illustration by means of case studies. cidence of adverse reactions and drug interac- tio is high, and suitable clients are not difficult to find.

Classroom discussion may be stimulated by consideration of questions such as the following:

1 □ What are the different types of adverse reactions to drugs? Describe and explain what is meant by the following:
- **a.** Side effects
- **b.** Allergic reactions
- **c.** Idiosyncratic reactions
- **d.** Chain reactions
- **e.** Cumulative reactions
- **f.** Tolerance and dependence

2 □ What are the different types of mechanisms responsible for drug interactions? Give one specific example of each mechanism.

3 □ What drugs would pose special difficulties for the following patients?
- **a.** Depressed clients with beer or wine intake (MAO inhibitors)
- **b.** Patients on limited fluid intake, *i.e.*, 1200 ml per day (amoxicillin, sulfonamides)
- **c.** Adolescent clients with high calcium intake (tetracycline and tetracycline-type antibiotics)
- **d.** Heavy smokers being treated for bronchospasm related to chronic obstructive pulmonary disease (theophylline derivatives)
- **e.** Clients with an increased rate of gastric motility (enteric-coated preparations)
- **f.** Epileptics on phenobarbital (griseofulvin)
- **g.** Patients on phenylbutazone who develop a thromboembolic phenomenon (warfarin)

Evaluation Examples (Test Items)

MINICARE STUDY

Assign a written report on adverse reactions to drugs or drug interactions in a client who has been cared for by the student. Ask students to list data substantiating the problem, analyze the data, state the nursing diagnosis, and establish a plan to ameliorate the problem. If the student has had an opportunity to carry out the nursing care plan, ask for an evaluation based on criteria developed during the initial planning stage.

ESSAY QUESTION

1. Explain one mechanism by which a drug interaction may occur. Give two specific drugs that interact with each other by this mechanism or whose actions would be affected by this mechanism.

MULTIPLE CHOICE ITEMS

1. The likelihood of cumulative toxicity from a drug is
- *1. Inversely related to the therapeutic index
- 2. Directly related to the margin of safety
- 3. Independent of either margin of safety or therapeutic index
- 4. Inversely related to the degree to which the drug enters inactive tissue reservoirs

2. The identification of adverse reactions to medication is usually incomplete until the drug in question has been in use for at least
- 1. 1 year
- 2. 5 years
- *3. 10 years
- 4. 50 years

3. Iatrogenic is best defined as
- 1. Harmful or undesirable
- *2. Arising from the treatment
- 3. Persistent despite the treatment
- 4. Innate in the illness

4. Definitions of toxicity include
- a. Harmful symptoms arising from excessive dosage
- b. Any harm caused by a drug
- c. Changes in symptoms that occur as therapeutic effect is established
- *1. a, b
- 2. b, c
- 3. a, c
- 4. All of the above

5. Side effects are best defined as
- 1. Helpful effects of drugs other than the specific purpose for which the drug was prescribed
- 2. Harmful effects of drugs incidental to the specific purpose for which the drug was prescribed
- *3. Effects of the drug other than the specific purpose for which the drug was prescribed, both helpful and harmful
- 4. Effects of a drug exerted at sites other than the site at which the desired therapeutic effect occurs

6. Select the answer that best describes statements a and b:
- a. Tolerance produces no signs or symptoms other than a relative unresponsiveness to normal doses of a drug.
- b. Withdrawal is an iatrogenic condition that occurs when a drug on which a client is dependent is withdrawn.
- 1. a and b are both true and a helps to explain b
- *2. a and b are both true but a does not help to explain b
- 3. a is true and b is false and a helps to explain the falsity of b
- 4. both a and b are false

7. The client is receiving Maalox (magnesium and aluminum hydroxides) four to six times a day. Which antibiotic should be avoided?

*1. Tetracycline
2. Ampicillin
3. Amoxicillin
4. Erythromycin

8. Griseofulvin has been prescribed for the client's severe ringworm infection. If the client reports being on an additional medication, which of the following would seriously affect the use of griseofulvin?

1. Atropine
2. Erythromycin
3. Multivitamins
*4. Phenobarbital

9. The client is receiving methotrexate for acute lymphocytic leukemia. In your teaching plan you would stress that the client should not take

1. Multivitamins
*2. Acetylsalicylic acid
3. Prednisone
4. Warfarin

10. Isocarboxazid (Marplan) is being used by a depressed client. In doing a diet history, the nurse should be concerned if the patient reported an intake of

a. Cheddar cheese
b. Apricots
c. Pepperoni
d. Chocolate
e. Tomatoes

1. a, b, e
*2. a, c, d
3. b, c, d
4. b, d, e
5. All of the above

11. Use of phenylbutazone and tolbutamide simultaneously might cause

1. Hyperglycemia
2. Hyponatremia
*3. Hypoglycemia
4. Hypernatremia
5. Hypokalemia

12. A complication of long-term diphenylhydantoin therapy is anemia. This is related to an interaction mechanism during

1. Absorption
2. Distribution
*3. Biotransformation
4. Excretion

13. Penicillin serum levels will be higher and more sustained if the drug is administered concurrently with

1. Potassium
2. Phenelzine
3. Phenobarbital
*4. Probenicid

14. When antiemetics are prescribed on a PRN basis to reduce nausea and encourage eating, they are best administered

1. When nausea occurs
2. Before meals, if the client is anorexic or nauseated
*3. Before meals regardless of whether the client is anorexic or nauseated at that time
4. After meals when nausea is most likely

15. Clients with postural hypotension should be cautioned to

1. Remain in bed until all vertigo ceases
*2. Move slowly and arise gradually
3. Practice ambulating independently to increase ability to walk without staggering
4. Restrict fluids to decrease the likelihood of motion sickness

16. Nursing measures to relieve itching include

a. Warning the client not to scratch
b. Keeping the area that itches cool
c. Providing interesting activities for the client

1. a, b
*2. b, c
3. a, c
4. All of the above

17. A food that is laxative in effect is

1. Blackberries
*2. Pears
3. Tea
4. Strawberries

10 Interactions between Food and Medications

Pharmacologic Properties of Food
- *Toxins*
- *Protectants*
- *Nursing Management*

Food Additives
- *Safety*
- *Nursing Management*

Alteration of Drug Effect by Food
- *Modification of Drug Pharmacokinetics*
- *Modification of Drug Action*
- *Nursing Management*

Nutritional Changes Induced by Medications
- *Drugs Influencing Gastrointestinal Function*
- *Other Therapeutic Agents*
- *Epidemiology of Drug-Induced Nutritional Deficiency*
- *Nursing Management*

Chapter 10 enhances the student's understanding of potential and actual food–drug interactions. The student is introduced to natural and artificial components of food that are pharmacologically active. The mechanisms underlying food–drug interactions are delineated. A final section describes common nutritional deficiencies caused by drugs. This chapter emphasizes the physiologic effects of food–drug interactions in people. The role of the professional nurse is presented as that of client advocate and consumer educator to promote safe and effective health practices relating to foods and drugs taken concurrently.

Through the study of this chapter, the student may develop the following concepts:

1 □ Natural toxins are found in many food sources, both plant and animal.
2 □ In most foods, toxins are present in such low concentrations that they are degraded about as rapidly as they are ingested.
3 □ It is sometimes possible to remove enough toxin from a very poisonous substance that it can be subsequently used as food.
4 □ When dangerous levels of toxins cannot easily be removed from a substance, the material is not normally classified as food.
5 □ Certain foods are popularly considered to confer health benefits on their consumers. These reputations may or may not be validated by research.
6 □ When taken to excess, even beneficial nutrients can cause adverse reactions.
7 □ The healthiest diet is one that includes a wide variety of foods taken in moderate amounts.
8 □ Individuals with food allergies should avoid consuming the specific substances to which they react adversely.
9 □ Information about pharmacologic properties of plant and animal tissues is most likely to be obtained from experts in the fields of pharmacognosy, conservation, botany, or horticulture.
10 □ Physicians, nurses, dieticians, and nutritionists should work together to assist clients to avoid adverse reactions to foods and harmful food–drug interactions.
11 □ Nurses can assist clients to ameliorate certain health problems through manipulation of the diet.
12 □ Many substances added to foods during processing are potentially harmful or of unproven safety.
13 □ In "developed" countries, problems of overnutrition are more common than are nutritional deficiencies.
14 □ Vitamin A toxicity is a fairly common problem of overnutrition.
15 □ Certain food additives can cause acute, life-threatening allergic reactions.
16 □ The presence or absence of food in the gastrointestinal tract markedly influences the absorption of many medications.
17 □ Foods may influence the action of drugs by altering either their pharmacokinetics or their pharmacodynamics.
18 □ Food components can form undigestible complexes with medications, if they mix in the GI tract.
19 □ Charcoal (in charbroiled foods) can adsorb drugs and prevent their absorption.
20 □ Dissolution of drugs proceeds faster in a warm medium than in a cold one.
21 □ Certain types of enteric coatings for medicinal tablets dissolve prematurely in the stomach if the *p*H of stomach contents is elevated.
22 □ Choice of foods can alter the *p*H of urine because some foods leave an acid "ash" following metabolism, while others leave an alkaline "ash."
23 □ Lowering the *p*H of urine promotes excretion of alkaline salts whereas raising its *p*H promotes excretion of acid salts.
24 □ Certain food–drug interactions can be life-threatening.
25 □ When monoamine oxidase inhibitors are prescribed, the client must avoid foods rich in tyrosine.
26 □ Certain nutrients act as antagonists of certain drugs.
27 □ When nutrients influence the action of a drug, they should not be excluded wholly from the diet, but their intake should be kept as uniform as possible so that the dose of medication can be stabilized.
28 □ Food–drug interaction can involve alteration of complex enzymatic metabolic processes.
29 □ Some drugs affect nutrition by a direct effect on gastrointestinal function. They may correct GI malfunction or they may cause a pathological malfunction of that system.

30 □ Anorexia, nausea, and vomiting are very common side effects of therapeutic drugs.
31 □ Medications can affect nutrition by interacting with nutrients in the same ways that they interact with other drugs.
32 □ Food–drug interactions occur more frequently in areas where "modern" medicine is practiced than in more "backward" parts of the world.
33 □ Many risk factors predispose an individual to food–drug interactions. These include poor nutritional state, presence of disease, physiologic need for nutrients, and genetic inheritance.
34 □ Medical risk factors for food–drug interaction include the nature of the prescribed drug regimen, the nature of the illness, the duration of both illness and drug treatment, the use of dialysis, and the physician's knowledge and skill in the field of nutrition.

Teaching Strategies

1 □ Assign students to small groups of three to five members for work on projects. Assign each group an activity on which it will report back to the class. Activities might include such topics as the following:

a. Investigate the types of vegetation in your area. As resources, consult with local conservation offices, horticulturists, or botanists. Ask about plants known to be poisonous when ingested, and about wild plants that are appropriate to use as foods. Be sure to obtain information about differentiating edible from toxic mushrooms.

b. Investigate herbs used as medications or as foods in your area. Consult with individuals or groups interested in "natural" foods, or with botanists or horticulturists. Collect as much information as possible about plants used to make herbal teas. Look up these substances in books dealing with toxicology to ascertain whether they contain potentially harmful substances. (*Hint*: Camomile, used to make herbal tea, causes adverse reactions in certain people.)

c. Identify various cultural influences on the selection of foods and beverages. Do food avoidance or prohibitions reflect beliefs or stigmas of particular groups? Are any related to genetic traits in the populations involved? Are these practices considered appropriate in the light of present knowledge about food characteristics? (Some groups that might be selected are Jews, Amish, Hindus, or Chinese.)

d. Devise a 2-hour educational program on food–drug interactions that would be suitable for presentation to a hospital or nursing home nursing staff. Include as examples drug regimens commonly prescribed in the institution you select. Explore techniques for instructing clients on oral medications.

e. Develop a "nutrition–drug therapy plan" suitable for use by nurses caring for clients of all ages in a rehabilitation center. Assume that clients are receiving long-term therapy for musculoskeletal injuries, chronic diseases of the aged, cancer, and/or congenital conditions such as cystic fibrosis, hemophilia, or phenylketonuria. Include in your plan specific foods or food additives that should be avoided by certain individuals in your clientele.

2 □ From institutionalized clients assigned to members of the class for clinical experience, choose individuals with drug regimens and diets that pose risk of food–drug interaction. During class time, divide the class into groups and present to each data related to one of these clients. Allow time for the development of a nursing care plan dealing with problems related to the diet, the medical regimen, or both. Have each group lead class discussion on its client situation.

Evaluation Examples (Test Items)

ESSAY QUESTIONS

1. Explain a mechanism by which food can influence the effect of enteric-coated tablets.

2. Identify at least four dietary minerals. Describe two examples of alteration of drug action by these minerals.

3. Discuss briefly how the presence of food in the intestinal tract may influence the effects of oral medications.

4. Identify two drug-induced nutritional deficiencies. Discuss briefly what should be done in each situation to promote optimum nutrition and therapeutic drug effect.

MULTIPLE CHOICE ITEMS

1. When should ion exchange resin (*e.g.*, cholestyramine) be administered?

1. At mealtime to facilitate absorption
2. Before meals when bile acid levels in the gut are lowest
3. After meals when bile is likely to be present in the gut
*4. Between meals to prevent adsorption of food nutrients

2. A food substance that can cause skeletal abnormalities in susceptible people is

1. Tea
2. Cyanide
*3. Lathyrogen
4. Thiaminase

3. Foods containing high quantities of tyrosine include all of the following *except*

1. Aged cheese
2. Beer
*3. Cereals
4. Chocolate
5. Salami

4. Foods containing tyrosine should be avoided by persons on long-term therapy using the drug(s)

1. L-dopa
2. Major tranquilizers
3. Cholestyramine
*4. Monoamineoxidase inhibitors

5. To maximize absorption of iron supplements, these drugs may be administered

a. With vitamin C
b. With milk products
c. On an empty stomach
d. With fruit juice

1. a, b, d
2. b, c
*3. a, c, d
4. a, b, c
5. d only

TRUE AND FALSE STATEMENTS

_T_ **1.** Enteric-coated tablets are best administered on an empty stomach.

_F_ **2.** Tetracycline antibiotics should be given with food to minimize stomach irritation.

_F_ **3.** To reduce the risk of digitalis toxicity, clients receiving cardiotonic drugs should use foods rich in sodium.

_T_ **4.** Hot foods and beverages taken with medication facilitate the dissolution of drugs.

11 Psychological Aspects of Drug Therapy

Behavioral Responses to Drugs
- *Attitudes*
- *Motivation*
- *Meaning Attached to Drugs*
- *Power of Suggestion*
- *Type of Illness*
- *The Nurse's Behavioral Response*
- *Behavioral Factors*

Nursing Management

Chapter 11 identifies psychologic factors that have a positive or negative effect on drug therapy. It helps the student to understand the uniqueness of each client's response to taking medications. The attitudes and values of the nurse and the client that interact to enhance or lower drug effectiveness are identified. The student is helped to identify behavioral responses that might affect drug therapy. The nurse's role in increasing or decreasing drug effectiveness is identified.

The student should understand the following concepts:

1 □ Each person has a unique response to drug therapy as a result of genetic, cultural, familial, socioeconomic, and educational factors.

2 □ Persons are not usually aware of values and attitudes that motivate drug-taking behavior.

3 The meaning attached to drugs is different for each person and influences the response to drug treatment.

4 □ The emotional state of the client helps to determine the client's response to drug therapy.

5 □ The family plays an important part in the client's compliance with a drug regime, as do the benefits of the client's maintaining the sick role.

6 □ The response of the patient with a chronic or terminal illness is different from that of the patient with an acute, short-term illness.

7 □ The nurse can enhance or decrease drug effectiveness through knowledge, skill, and attitude.

Teaching Strategies

1 □ Classroom discussion might include students' personal experiences at home or in the hospital setting. It should focus on identification of students' values and attitudes toward drugs that might arouse strong emotional responses. These might include vitamins, aspirin, Motrin, codeine for menstrual discomfort, Premarin during menopause, contraceptive drugs for teenagers, high dosages of narcotics to control pain of the terminally ill or postsurgical client, or use of alcohol and street drugs.

2 □ Small group discussions might focus on students identifying their own cultural backgrounds and their influence on drug-taking behaviors.

- **a.** In a small group, students could share personal experiences of hospitalization and their perception of the nurse's attitude when administering a medication to them. In what way did the nurse's behavior enhance or lower drug effectiveness?
- **b.** Identify the number of drugs the student has taken over the past 6 months. Is this a usual patttern? Compare this with their family's usual pattern of drug use.
- **c.** What stereotypes do students have of how people from different cultural backgrounds respond to drug taking? Discuss instances when these responses were different from what was expected.

3 □ A film or filmstrip such as the following could be shown:

- **a.** Person-to-Person Relationships (Film, National Audio Visual Center, Rental or Sales Branch, Washington, DC 20409; explores attitudes and skills in getting along with each other.
- **b.** Interactions for Study (Filmstrip, Concept Media, 1500 Adams Ave., Costa Mesa, CA 92626); illustrates various types of nonverbal communication.

Evaluation Examples (Test Items)

MULTIPLE CHOICE ITEMS

1. When administering drugs to a client, the nurse should be aware of

a. The meaning that taking drugs has for the client
b. The degree of motivation
c. Genetics
d. Intensity of responses

1. a
*2. a, b
3. b, d
4. c, d
5. All of the above

2. When following a drug regimen, the client who uses the sick role for secondary gains would be most likely to

1. Take the drug and feel better
2. Disregard the family's attitude
*3. Take the drug, but develop other symptoms
4. Feel better if the nurse is reassuring

3. The nurse can best have a positive effect on the client's responses to drugs by

1. Using the resources of the health team
2. Having a knowledge of drugs
*3. Having a positive attitude toward drug therapy
4. Understanding families
5. Understanding disease processes

12 Cultural Aspects of Drug Therapy

Ethnomedicine
- *Black Americans*
- *Hispanic Americans*
- *Asian Americans*
- *Native Americans*
- *White Americans of European Descent*

Ethnopharmacology
- *Preparation and Use of Herbs*
- *Applications of Ethnopharmacology*

Nursing Management

Chapter 12 provides the student with the opportunity to survey the five major cultural groups existing in the United States today. The beliefs commonly shared by these populations are discussed in relation to health and illness practices, as well as to remedies used in the prevention and treatment of illness.

The science of ethnopharmacology is presented as the vehicle for the study of the different cultures. It allows for the exploration of folk practices in the traditional use of medicinal plants and for consideration of the legitimate use of botanic drugs within the cultural context.

The information provided in this chapter is intended to enhance the ability of the nurse to incorporate knowledge about significant health beliefs and traditional folk practices into planning for patient care needs. This knowledge base has the potential to facilitate social and psychologic support for patients interacting with the Western health-care delivery system by accommodating traditional beliefs and alternative ways of healing into current nursing practice.

Concepts presented reflect similarities and differences among the populations discussed. Concepts the students may develop are the following:

1 □ The significance placed on certain disease-related problems may be culture-specific.
2 □ Cultural differences in health and illness beliefs influence the ability of a person to react to, and take action to remediate, the problem.
3 □ Beliefs about the nature of humankind and its ability to effect change or control over its environment influence health and illness practices.
4 □ Several factors determine the health and illness practices of ethnic groups: cross-cultural influences, socioeconomic status, language facility, strength and significance of kinship ties, and degree to which one accepts the beliefs and values of the dominant culture.
5 □ Recognition of the active ingredients contained in plants is essential to the determination of the efficacy of herbal remedies used in traditional folk practices.
6 □ The active ingredients in many of the prescribed medicines used today are natural products.
7 □ Traditional rules for plant collection, use, and storage in ethnopharmacology are specific and intended to promote safe use.

Teaching Strategies

Several methods could be used to promote exploration of cross-cultural similarities and differences. These may include the following:

1 □ Classroom discussion might include using a seminar format to facilitate sharing personal experiences related to family folk practices.
2 □ Panel discussion might involve community health-care providers who represent the various cultural groups discussed.
3 □ Assign students to interview community members from the various cultural groups and present their findings to the class in a panel discussion.
4 □ Invite people who practice alternative or traditional methods of healing to discuss their beliefs in the classroom. These could include a *curandero*, medicine man, or acupuncturist.
5 □ Present a patient situation for discussion that represents the potential for conflict between traditional values and Western, holistic health-care delivery. For example, discuss the beliefs of the native American Indian and speculate about the potential for conflict between cultural beliefs and current medical practice.
6 □ Assign selected students to observe health-care delivery in a neighborhood health center in which specific cultural groups interface with current medical practices. Students should interview various providers to explore the nature of traditional beliefs seen.

Evaluation Examples (Test Items)

MULTIPLE CHOICE ITEMS

1. Among black Americans, traditional beliefs about health and illness reflect
- *1. A belief that illness is a result of natural causes
- 2. A belief that people are responsible for solving their own problems to restore harmony
- 3. A belief that the only person with the power to cure is God
- 4. A belief that healing can occur only through the spirits

2. Hispanic beliefs regarding the nature of illness include all of the following *except*
- 1. Dislocation of body parts can result in illness
- *2. Misuse of ceremonial rituals may cause illness

3. Envy or intense emotional state may result in illness
4. Body imbalances may cause illness

3. Maintaining a balance between hot and cold is characteristic of which Puerto Rican belief system?
1. Holistic
2. Personalistic
*3. Naturalistic

4. Chinese physicians use the practice of glossoscopy to diagnose body imbalances. This practice refers to
1. Consultation with a spiritual healer
2. Palpation of deep and superficial pulses
3. Listening and smelling
*4. Inspection of external appearance

5. American Indian health and illness beliefs include which of the following?
a. Inclusion of the total family in diagnosing a condition
b. Respect for the universe supersedes all other concerns in maintaining health and harmony
c. One must deal with the illness rather than with the causative external event
d. Illness is believed to be purposeful
1. a, c, d
2. b, c
*3. a, d
4. All of the above

6. Collection of herbs by Native Americans follows which of these beliefs?
1. Plants with a western exposure are most potent
2. Plants that receive the late afternoon rays are best
3. Springtime is considered to be the best time to harvest herbs for drying
*4. Collection of plants in the early morning is most efficacious

7. The most common form of preparation of dried plants for medicinal purposes is
*1. A tisane
2. A maceration
3. An infusion
4. A decoction

8. Which of the following plants have been used to treat malignant conditions?
a. American mandrake (*Podophyllum peltatum*)
b. Rauwolfia (*Rauwolfia serpentina*)
c. Meadow saffron (*Colchicum autumnale*)
d. American hellebore (*Veratrum viride*)
1. a, b
*2. a, c
3. b, c
4. a, c, d
5. All of the above

9. Medicinal plants used for soothing and pain-reducing qualities include all of the following except
1. Opium poppy (*Papaver somniferum*)
2. Henbane (*Hyoscyamus niger*)
3. Common lettuce (*Lactuce virosa*)
*4. Periwinkle (*Catharanthus roseus*)

UNIT THREE: ADMINISTRATION OF MEDICATIONS

13 Basic Principles of Medication

Role Functions Related to Drug Therapy
- *Pharmacist*
- *Physician, Dentist, and Veterinarian*
- *Paraprofessionals*
- *Nurses*
- *Trends in the Assignment of Role Functions*

Nursing Management
- *Nursing Implications*
- *Nursing Process*

Delivery of Drug Doses
- *The Right Drug*
- *The Right Dose*
- *The Right Client*
- *The Right Route*
- *The Right Time*

Nursing Management of Drug Therapy for Institutionalized Clients
- *Medication Procedures Used in Institutions*

Medication Errors
- *Causes*
- *Reporting an Error*

Chapter 13 introduces the student to knowledge basic to the pharmacologic aspects of nursing care. The chapter describes current role functions of health professionals in drug therapy in relation to their historical evolution and the current trends toward expansion of responsibilities of nurses, pharmacists, and paraprofessionals. Aspects of pharmacology pertinent to each step of the nursing process are discussed. The student is introduced to procedures commonly used for delivery of drug doses and safety measures to prevent medication errors.

Through the study of this chapter, students may develop the following concepts:

1 □ Role functions of health professionals are constantly evolving; the trend is for increased delegation of tasks previously reserved for physicians to other health-care providers.
2 □ Some role functions related to medicinal use of drugs are assigned by law to various health professionals: physicians and dentists may perform all role functions (but most frequently diagnose and prescribe), pharmacists compound and dispense drugs, nurses manage drug regimens and deliver drug doses, and paraprofessionals perform narrowly delineated functions pertinent to their area of expertise.
3 □ Role functions of health professionals vary somewhat from setting to setting.
4 □ Pharmacology has implications for professional practice in every step of the nursing process: assessment, analysis, diagnosis, planning, implementation, and evaluation.
5 □ Drug effects are influenced by many factors, including absorption, distribution, metabolism and excretion of the drug, and the client's state of health and allergic sensitivity.
6 □ Careful assessment, analysis, and decision making by the nurse are required for optimal management of medicinal drug regimens.
7 □ Accuracy in delivery of drug doses requires careful attention to five factors: drug, dose, client, route of administration, and time.
8 □ Procedures for delivery of drug doses may vary in their details but must be based on principles conducive to safety and efficacy.
9 □ The development of good procedural habits promotes accuracy and efficiency in the delivery of drug doses.
10 □ Adherence to rules and guidelines promotes safety and efficacy in most situations but may pose risks in unusual circumstances; sound judgment is required for optimum care in individual situations.
11 □ Client education regarding drug use is an important aspect of nursing care.

Teaching Strategies

Assignment of learning experiences depends on the placement of pharmacology in the nursing curriculum. If this content is presented early, field experiences will be primarily observational. Practice in the skills laboratory in medication administration may profitably be coordinated with the study of Unit Three. If students are already involved in the care of clients, they may begin the integration of this knowledge into clinical practice immediately. Other class activities might include the following:

1 □ Allot class time for discussion of student observation experiences outlined in the Learning Experiences in the text. When medication practices in settings used for clinical laboratory are considered, point out the relation of administrative policies such as staffing patterns to procedures used in the nursing units and in the pharmacy.
2 □ Invite pharmacists, physicians, respiratory therapists, and other professionals involved in drug regimens to talk with the students about ways in which nurses and other health professionals may collaborate to enhance the safety and efficacy of drug therapy.
3 □ Assign selected students to observe health professionals at work to determine the degree to which their work involves knowledge and skills relating to pharmacology. Include as many of the following cate-

gories as possible: physicians, pharmacists, nurses (in various settings), laboratory technicians, x-ray technicians, respiratory therapists, and ward and pharmacy clerks. During class discussion, consider the need to understand the actions and effects of poisonous substances such as test reagents as well as those of medicinal drugs. Compare and contrast the functions of professional and vocational nurses in various settings such as hospitals, skilled nursing facilities, health-related facilities, mental health settings, and community health agencies.

4 □ Discuss in class the role that standard procedures and personal habits play in promoting efficiency and safety in the delivery of drug doses in institutional settings (hospitals and nursing homes). Drawing on student observations and your own experience, discuss distractions impinging on practitioners in these settings during administration of medications.

5 □ Discuss laws regulating the role functions of health professionals in relation to drug therapy in your state. Compare the provisions of these regulations with the national trend of expanding the role of the nurse.

6 □ Review the sample medication procedures outlined in the text, explaining the implications of the rationale for each nursing action. Compare and contrast the use of medication cards and carts, identifying the strengths and weaknesses of each method for administering drugs.

7 □ Divide the class into groups of four to eight students. Assign each group to develop a procedure for delivery of drug doses in one of the following situations:

a. Imagine you are the nurse in a summer camp in which one hundred children 10 to 15 years old are residents. The staff includes 20 counselors 16 to 22 years old and 12 adults. What policies and procedures would be appropriate for administration of medicinal drugs needed by this population? If the administration of some drug substances are to be delegated to people other than the nurse (*e.g.*, oxygen given to victims of near-drowning administered by the waterfront director or lifeguard), what should be done to promote the safety and efficacy of these practices?

b. Imagine you are a nurse acting as a consultant for house parents and counselors who administer community residences for the retarded. What policies and procedures would be appropriate for administration of medicinal drugs needed by the residents if there are insufficient funds to hire nurses to perform this function?

c. Imagine that you have been requested to act as a consultant for the staff of a shelter for homeless men. They wish advice on medication practices for the residence. Most of the residents have a history of alcoholism and there is a high incidence of tuberculosis and liver impairment. The facility is administered by a Catholic priest but otherwise is staffed entirely by volunteers. Devise a procedure for delivery of drug doses. What policies would you advise to control drugs in this setting?

8 □ Use anecdotes to illustrate the role of the professional nurse in adapting guidelines and protocols required by individual circumstances. Emphasize the importance of sound rationale and critical judgment when decisions to depart from established procedure are considered.

Evaluation Examples (Test Items)

ESSAY QUESTIONS

1. Briefly discuss the role functions related to drug therapy of physicians, pharmacists, professional nurses, and vocational nurses.

2. List and discuss briefly the knowledge and skills related to pharmacology required in the steps of the nursing process: assessment, diagnosis, planning, implementation, and evaluation.

3. Briefly compare and contrast medication procedures using medication cards with those using medication carts, including both strengths and weaknesses of each.

SHORT ANSWER QUESTIONS

1. Name the *five rights* that must be considered when delivering drug doses.

2. List five questions you would ask of a client while taking a drug history.

3. Define the verbs "compound," "dispense," and "prescribe" as they relate to drug therapy.

MULTIPLE CHOICE ITEMS

1. Legally, the right to prescribe drugs is usually limited to physicians and

1. Nurses
*2. Dentists
3. Optometrists
4. Pharmacists
5. All of the above

2. The delivery of most drug doses to clients in hospital settings is carried out by

1. Physicians
*2 Nurses
3. Pharmacists
4. Pharmacy technicians

3. For most drugs administered medicinally, a dose may deviate from the prescribed dose by as much as

1. 0%—no deviation is allowed
2. 1%
3. 5%
*4. 10%

4. For most drugs, the time required for elimination of residues from the body in a normally healthy client is about

1. 6 hours
2. 2 days

3. 1 week
*4. 2 weeks

5. In which of the following situations are medications commonly used without the involvement of health-care professionals? (Check all that apply.)

1. Use of legend drugs
*2. Use of over-the-counter drugs
*3. Use of folk remedies
4. Medicinal use of narcotics
*5. Therapy by an herbalist

14
Special Skills Related to Drug Administration

Storage and Handling of Drugs
Preservation
Containers
Childproof Caps
Tamper-proof Packaging
Storage in the Home
Storage in Institutions
Insulin
Learning the Language
Physicians' Orders for Medication
Computation of Drug Doses
The Metric System
Household Measures
Apothecary Measures
Conversion from One Measurement System to Another
Computation of Doses
Preparing of Solutions
Preparing Fractional Doses from Solid Drugs
Verifying Computed Dosage
Occupational Hazards Related To Drug Administration
Chemical Dependence
Adverse Reaction to Toxic Substances
Antibiotic-resistant Infections
Blood-borne Infections
Allergy
Nursing Implications

Chapter 14 presents material on proper drug storage, terminology used for drug orders (including abbreviations), the elements of a prescription or drug order, systems of measurement used in drug therapy, and computation of drug doses. Through Learning Experiences, the student may be introduced to the facilities available in health-care settings and institutions for the preparation of medications.

Among the concepts students may develop in this chapter are the following:

1 □ Environmental control is necessary to prevent premature deterioration of drug preparations.
2 □ Legible labels on drug containers are necessary for identification of the contents of the containers.
3 □ Drug supplies must be kept in a secure place to prevent inappropriate use by unauthorized persons.
4 □ Written orders or prescriptions from the physician are necessary because they present clear and specific directions on drug therapy.
5 □ Accuracy must be developed to determine safe computation of drug doses.

Students may also develop skill in the mathematical processes involved in converting drug doses from one system of measurement to another, and in computing drug doses.

Teaching Strategies

The degree to which the content of this chapter can be integrated into clinical practice depends on the placement of the material in the curriculum. If pharmacology is taught prior to the initial institutional experiences, some of the learning experiences will be difficult to arrange. Some laboratory practice (within the school setting) in computation of doses and manipulation of equipment used to measure drug doses would be valuable if this is the case. The following are examples of class activities:

1 □ Exhibit samples of drugs that have deteriorated as a result of prolonged or inappropriate storage (*e.g.*, aspirin tablets that are chipped or broken because of mechanical trauma, tablets eroded by dissolution from atmospheric humidity, color changes in aged tablets, or aspirin old enough to smell of vinegar). Discuss clinical problems that could result from use of such drugs (*e.g.*, inaccurate doses, failure of therapeutic effect, adverse reactions).
2 □ Discuss the financial impact of wasting drug preparations on the cost of health care. Quote local prices of specific drugs when administered in institutional settings, and when purchased from a drug store.
3 □ Work on conversion and computation problems in class or in the school laboratory. Demonstrate the "pouring" of drug doses, using equipment in common use in local clinical settings. Allow the students to manipulate and examine the equipment.

Evaluation Examples (Test Items)

ESSAY QUESTION

1. Describe the special precautions taken when doses of controlled drugs such as opiates are prepared in institutional settings.

SHORT ANSWER QUESTION

Define the following:

ac	tid
ad lib	stat
bid	ss
gtt	tr
hs	ung
IM	ASA
IV	MOM
OS	SSKI
qd	SSE
PRN	MO

MULTIPLE CHOICE ITEMS

1. Most drugs should be stored in an environment that is

1. Cold and dark
*2. Cool and dry
3. Warm and dry
4. Light and airy

2. Insulin should be allowed to reach room temperature before it is administered because

1. Cold insulin is absorbed more slowly than warm insulin
2. Higher doses are required when cold insulin is used
*3. Changes in fatty tissue at injection sites are more likely to develop when cold insulin is used
4. Administration of cold insulin causes pain at the injection site

3. Stock drugs are those

1. Derived from tissues of cattle
2. Normally available immediately from the institution pharmacy
3. Normally found on the shelves of all nursing units in the institution
*4. Dispensed in quantity in a single container from which doses are poured for a number of clients

4. A complete medication order should *always* inclue

a. The name of the drug to be given and the dose
b. The number of tablets or milliliters or other quantities to be given
c. The route to be used
d. The clock hours when the drug is to be given

*1. a, c
2. b, c
3. a, d
4. b, d
5. All of the above

5. Which of the following is *not* an approved equivalent for the number of milligrams in one grain?

1. 60 mg
2. 64 mg
3. 65 mg
4. 66-2/3 mg
*5. 68 mg

UNIT FOUR: DRUGS USED FOR INFLAMMATIONS AND INFECTIONS

15
Major Antimicrobial Drugs

Introduction to Anti-infectives
Introduction to Antimicrobials
Characteristics of the Ideal Antimicrobial
The Use of Antimicrobials
Pharmacodynamics
Adverse Reactions
Treatment Failures
Nursing Management
Major Antimicrobial Drug Families
Sulfonamides
Beta-lactam Antibiotics
Aminoglycosides
Tetracyclines
Erythromycins
Chloramphenicol

Chapter 15 deals with antimicrobial drugs frequently used to prevent or treat bacterial infection. These treatment agents usually are administered systemically. Except for the topical preparations, which act locally, they are prescribed for a systemic effect.

Through the study of this chapter, students may develop the following concepts:

1 □ Antimicrobial drugs are curative; they help the body to eliminate the cause of infection.
2 □ All antimicrobial drugs have the potential for inducing adverse reactions.
3 □ Adverse reactions to antimicrobial drugs include allergic reactions, damage to rapidly dividing cells, kidney and liver impairment, damage to nerves (especially the eighth cranial nerve), bone and teeth defects, and superinfection.
4 □ Selection of the proper antimicrobial for treatment depends on the sensitivity of the microorganisms causing the infection, and on risk factors that influence client response to drugs.
5 □ When antimicrobials are recommended, the entire prescription should be taken as directed, even though the signs and symptoms of illness may have disappeared.
6 □ Excessive use of antimicrobial therapy stimulates the development of resistant strains of organisms and increases the likelihood of adverse reactions in clients receiving the drugs.
7 □ When needed, antimicrobial therapy should be instituted as early as possible to prevent the development of larger populations of pathogens.
8 □ Successful prevention or elimination of infection by antimicrobial therapy depends, in part, on the natural body defenses against infection.
9 □ The availability of effective antimicrobial drug agents does not eliminate the need for nursing measures to reduce the transmission of pathogens and to support the recovery process in persons with infections.
10 □ Pollution of the environment with antimicrobials increases the incidence of allergic hypersensitivity in clients and stimulates the development of resistant strains of organisms.
11 □ Clients receiving antimicrobials, especially sulfonamide drugs, should be well hydrated.
12 □ When administered intravenously, antimicrobials tend to irritate veins.
13 □ Clients exhibiting allergic hypersensitivity to some antibiotics may also exhibit cross sensitivity to related compounds.
14 □ Aqueous solutions of antibiotics tend to break down chemically with the passage of time and should be administered within the recommended time period after preparation; most require refrigeration.
15 □ Antimicrobial medication administered orally must be carefully timed in relation to meals because food may interfere with the action of the medications.
16 □ The administration of food containing lactobacilli helps to maintain a normal intestinal flora in clients receiving antimicrobial therapy.
17 □ Tetracyclines are not administered during pregnancy or to young persons whose teeth are in the process of formation.
18 □ Chloramphenicol is considered a drug of last resort to be used only in serious infections caused by organisms resistant to other antimicrobials.

Teaching Strategies

The use of antimicrobials is so pervasive in modern societies that examples illustrating the material in this chapter are plentiful. The instructor may draw on the personal experience of students, the histories of well clients, and the use of antimicrobials in health-care settings for examples.

□ Classroom discussion might consider such questions as the following:

a. How prevalent are infections among clients in local health-care institutions?
b. Of the infections found in institutionalized clients, what proportion is nosocomial?
c. How often is chloramphenicol prescribed for clients in local health-care institutions? For what conditions is the drug used?

d. How often are antimicrobial drugs prescribed prophylactically? In what clinical situations?
e. Have antimicrobial-resistant infections been found in local health-care institutions? What was (is being) done to eliminate these pathogens?
f. When clients receive prescriptions for antimicrobial drugs, what instructions do they receive about the treatment regimen and the self-care needed during the course of treatment?

Evaluation Examples (Test Items)

ESSAY QUESTIONS

1. Identify and describe briefly at least three mechanisms by which systemic antimicrobial drugs affect microorganisms.

2. Identify and describe briefly at least two mechanisms by which an organism may develop resistance to a given antimicrobial.

SHORT ANSWER QUESTION

Define or explain the meaning of the following terms

Spectrum of activity	Antibiotic
Resistant organism	Anaphylaxis
Superinfection	Culture and sensitivity

MULTIPLE CHOICE ITEMS

1. Allergic hypersensitivity is stimulated most often when antimicrobial drugs are administered
*1. Topically
2. Orally
3. By inhalation
4. By injection

2. Allergic reactions to antimicrobial drugs are most apt to be manifested when the drugs are administered
1. Topically
2. Orally
3. By inhalation
*4. By injection

3. The most serious allergic reaction to antimicrobials is
1. Urticaria
*2. Anaphylaxis
3. Inflammation at the injection site
4. Superinfection

4. At 10 PM a child with a crush injury to the hand is transferred to your unit from the surgical recovery room. An antibiotic order has been written that specifies a dosage well above the usual dosage range for the child's size. You should
1. Delay giving the drug until the physician's morning rounds, when the dosage can be verified
2. Contact the physician immediately to question the drug dosage
*3. Give the antibiotic because the nature of the injury requires treatment by high doses of antimicrobials
4. Give a dose of the antibiotic equal to the maximum recommended dose for the child's size

5. A diabetic client is admitted to your unit with a furuncle on the back of the neck. The physician has ordered a broad-spectrum antibiotic to be administered intravenously. You should give the antibiotic
1. Immediately
2. As soon as glucose balance has been assessed by a urine or blood test
*3. As soon as specimens of drainage from the furuncle have been taken for culture and sensitivity tests
4. After contacting the physician to verify the route for medication in this infection-prone patient

6. A young man being treated for an eye injury is receiving chloramphenicol systemically. When assessing him for any adverse reaction to the medication, you should monitor
1. Respirations and blood pressure
*2. Blood cell levels
3. Urinary output, BUN, creatine, and results of urinalysis
4. Liver enzymes

7. Several clients in your nursing home are receiving maintenance doses of sulfonamides to prevent urinary tract infections. Measures to reduce the risk of adverse reactions to the drugs include
a. As far as possible, reduce the incidence of urinary bladder catheterization so that the antibiotic may be discontinued
b. Teach clients and staff proper techniques of personal hygiene related to cleansing of the external genitalia to reduce the need for the drugs
c. Serve a quart of cranberry juice daily to each client receiving sulfonamides
*1. a, b
2. b, c
3. a, c
4. All of the above

8. When taking a health history from a client who is likely to receive tetracycline, it is most important to ask whether the client
1. Is allergic to penicillin
2. Has ever received tetracycline
3. Has a history of liver problems
*4. Is lactating, or might be pregnant (if a young woman)

16 Antimycobacterial Agents, Miscellaneous Antimicrobials, and Urinary Tract Antiseptics

Antimycobacterial Agents
- *Streptomycin*
- *Ethambutol*
- *Hydrochloride Isomazid*
- *Rifampin*
- *Para-aminosalicylic Acid*
- *Capreomycin*
- *Cycloserine*
- *Ethionamide*
- *Pyrazinamide*
- *Sulfoxone Sodium*

Nursing Management
- *Nursing Implications*
- *Nursing Process*

Miscellaneous Antimicrobials
- *Azthreonam*
- *Bacitracin*
- *Clindamycin*
- *Colistin*
- *Lincomycin*
- *Nitrofurazone*
- *Novabiocin*
- *Polymyxin B*
- *Spectinomycin*
- *Troleandomycin*
- *Sugar*

Nursing Management
- *Nursing Process*

Urinary Tract Antiseptics
- *Methenamine*
- *Nalidixic Acid*
- *Nitrofurantoin*
- *Phenazopyridine*
- *Trimethoprim*
- *Urine Acidifiers*

Nursing Management
- *Nursing Process*

Chapter 16 describes drugs used in the treatment of mycobacterial diseases (tuberculosis and leprosy), miscellaneous antimicrobials, and drugs used for urinary tract infection. Through the study of this chapter, students may develop the following concepts:

1 □ The goal of antimycobacterial drug treatment is arrest of the active infection; eradication of all pathogens is not a realistic goal.
2 □ Compliance with antimycobacterial drug regimens is difficult because treatment is long term (months or years), multiple drugs are prescribed, drugs are often taken several times a day, adverse reactions to the drugs can be serious, and repeated courses of drugs may be required if the infection becomes reactivated.
3 □ Prophylactic medication may be prescribed for clients at high risk for either initial or recurrent active mycobacterial infections.
4 □ Some antimicrobial drugs increase the need for specific nutrients, such as vitamins.
5 □ Therapeutic regimens for antimicrobial infections require frequent monitoring for response to treatment.
6 □ Discomfort at the site used for intramuscular injection of irritating drugs can be minimized by application of ice to the site before and after injection.
7 □ Antimicrobials that are poorly absorbed from the gastrointestinal tract are useful when administered orally for the treatment of infections affecting the intestinal tract.
8 □ It is not necessary always to know the exact mechanism of action of a drug; if it produces the desired effects without serious side effects, such a drug can be used empirically.
9 □ Women are at high risk for recurrent urinary tract infections.
10 □ Hygienic measures are as important as medication in the elimination and prevention of recurrent urinary tract infections.
11 □ Some urinary tract antiseptics require an acid urine to be effective.
12 □ Some anti-infective agents change the color of body fluids; client should be informed (and reassured) about these changes when drug therapy is initiated.

Teaching Strategies

This chapter may be assigned as part of the work required for a unit on the prevention and treatment of infectious disease. Alternatively, students may refer to it when caring for clients receiving drugs described in this part of the text.

□ Classroom or laboratory conference discussion might consider such questions as the following:

a. How prevalent are mycobacterial infections in the community?

b. How does present-day treatment of tuberculosis compare with treatment before the advent of antimicrobial drug therapy?

c. What antimicrobial drugs are prescribed most often by physicians in the local community or hospital? Are drugs listed in the text as "miscellaneous antimicrobials" utilized? What are the criteria for their use?

d. How prevalent is the long-term use of retention catheters in local health-care institutions? How prevalent are urinary tract infections in these institutions? What proportion of urinary tract infections are considered to be nosocomial?

Evaluation Examples (Test Items)

ESSAY QUESTIONS

1. List and discuss briefly specific assessment data that should be gathered relating to the client who is about to begin drug therapy for tuberculosis.

2. Outline and discuss briefly a program for teaching preventive measures to a female client with a history of recurrent urinary tract infections.

MULTIPLE CHOICE ITEMS

1. Realistic goals for drug therapy of people with mycobacterial infection are

a. Alleviation of acute symptoms
b. Arrest of the disease process
c. Elimination of live mycobacteria from the body
d. Prevention of spread of the infection to others

*1. a, b, d
2. b, c, d
3. a, c
4. All of the above

2. The mechanism of action of the urinary antiseptic methenamine is

1. Lowering of urine *p*H
2. Generation of ammonia within the urinary tract
*3. Generation of formaldehyde within the urinary tract
4. All of the above

3. Adult clients receiving methenamine to prevent urinary tract infection should be advised to

a. Limit fluids to 1500 ml/day to prevent dilution of the drugs in the urinary tract
b. Avoid the use of bubble bath or detergent bath salts
c. Use food that will lower urinary *p*H

1. a, b
*2. b, c
3. a, c
4. All of the above

17
Drugs Used to Treat Infections Caused by Viruses and Fungi

VIRAL INFECTIONS
Agents That Stimulate, Simulate, or Inhibit Host Responses to Viruses
Vaccines and Sera
Inducers of General Resistance
Anti-inflammatories
Antiviral Compounds
Acyclovir
Amantadine
Azidothymidine
Idoxuride
Ribavirin
Vidarabine
Nursing Management
Nursing Implications
Nursing Process
ANTIFUNGAL DRUGS
Superficial Fungal Infections
Astringents
Keratolytic Agents
Salts of Fatty Acids
Antiseptics
Antifungal Antibiotics
Nursing Management
Nursing Implications
Nursing Process
Systemic Fungal Infections
Amphoterecin B
Flucytosine
Ketoconazole and Micanazole
Nursing Management
Nursing Implications
Nursing Process

Chapter 17 deals with drug treatment of infections caused by viruses and fungi. Through the study of this chapter, the student may develop the following concepts:

1 □ Viruses multiply only within cells, using the mechanisms in the living cell for replication.
2 □ Drugs that affect viruses are likely to be harmful to the host's tissue cells.
3 □ At present, no safe broad-spectrum antiviral drug is available for the treatment of viral infections.
4 □ At present, the best pharmaceutical method of control of viral infections is preventive immunization.
5 □ Acceleration of the development of vaccines may increase the risk of adverse reactions in clients receiving the drugs.
6 □ Human immune globulin prevents the development of overt disease in susceptible persons who have been exposed to viruses by conferring a temporary passive immunity.
7 □ A natural body chemical, interferon, is under investigation as a broad-spectrum antiviral agent.
8 □ Antiviral compounds in present use are harmful to rapidly dividing cells and tend to be quite toxic.
9 □ Most fungal diseases tend to recur because they are caused by opportunistic organisms present on the skin or mucous membranes that multiply when conditions are conducive to their growth.
10 □ Many superficial fungal infections may be controlled through the use of astringent, keratolytic, and antiseptic agents.
11 □ The elimination of fungal microorganisms may require the administration of antifungal systemic drugs for a prolonged time.

Teaching Strategies

A comprehensive unit on infectious disease could incorporate the study of this chapter and Chapters 15, 16, 18, 19, 20 and 42. Nursing skills appropriate to such a unit include applications of heat or cold, injection technique, and medical asepsis (routine and isolation technique). Related content includes natural defenses against infection, the immune response, pathologic changes in severe infection, and current morbidity and mortality statistics related to infectious disease.

□ Topics for classroom discussions might include the following:

a. What difficulties are involved in developing systemic antiviral drugs?

b. What immunizations are recommended for normal infants? Are there local endemic diseases for which no immunization is recommended? Why is immunization not employed for these diseases? What is done to treat persons who contract these diseases?

c. What are the conditions that favor the development of opportunistic infections such as those caused by fungi?

Evaluation Examples (Test Items)

ESSAY QUESTIONS

1. Discuss the present state of drug treatment of viral infections. Include consideration of the following questions: What pharmaceutic agents are most effective in controlling viral infection? How do the number of drugs available for the treatment of active viral infection compare with the number available for the treatment of bacterial infection? What are the prospects for the future development of new agents through research? Identify at least one drug used for preventing viral infection, one used to treat active viral infections, and one substance currently under investigation for use as an antiviral drug.

2. A new mother asks you, "What immunizations should my baby have?" Outline the recommendations you would make about immunizations against viral disease. What information will the mother need about care of the infant following the administration of vaccines?

SHORT ANSWER QUESTIONS

1. List five measures you would recommend to reduce mild itching from "athlete's foot."

2. List five known adverse reactions to griseofulvin.

MULTIPLE CHOICE ITEMS

1. Toxic effects and side effects of vitamin C include
1. Alkalinization of the urine
*2. An increased risk of renal calculi
3. An increased tendency to bleed from small capillaries
4. None of the above—vitamin C has virtually no toxic or side effects

2. The infections that are usually the most difficult to treat because we have few effective drugs to combat them are those caused by
*1. Viruses
2. Gram-positive cocci
3. Gram-negative bacilli
4. Acid-fast bacilli

3. A drug used for the treatment of herpes simplex keratitis is
*1. Idoxuridine
2. Amantadine
3. Interferon
4. Methisazone

4. Routine immunization against one viral disease is no longer recommended because the disease appears to have been eradicated from earth. That disease is
1. Varicella
*2. Variola
3. Rubeola
4. Rubella
5. Infectious viral parotitis

5. Which of the following drugs is a keratolytic agent?
1. Alcohol
2. Gentian violet
3. Tannic acid
*4. Salicylanilide

6. The drug used most often for the treatment of thrush is
*1. Nystatin
2. Griseofulvin
3. Aluminum disulfide
4. Gentian violet

7. The drug administered to eliminate tinea organisms from the body is
1. Nystatin
*2. Griseofulvin
3. Aluminum disulfide
4. Gentian violet

8. A common household substance that acts as an astringent is
1. Vinegar
*2. Tea
3. Sodium bicarbonate
4. Salt solution

9. Clients receiving griseofulvin should decrease their consumption of
1. Tea
2. Sugar
3. Cigarettes
*4. Alcohol

10. Amphotericin B is usually administered
1. Orally
2. Topically
3. Intramuscularly
*4. Intravenously

11. The drug administered systemically to eliminate fungi from tissues such as toenails is
1. Alcohol
*2. Griseofulvin
3. Potassium permanganate
4. Nystatin

SITUATION-BASED MULTIPLE CHOICE ITEMS

Situation: Mr. MC, age 35 years, has developed a severe skin rash over the lower extremities and groin. This has been diagnosed as an extension and exacerbation of a chronic tinea pedis. (MC has had recurrent "athlete's foot" since his teens.) Griseofulvin (ultramicrosize) 250 mg bid has been ordered.

1. When taking a history from this client, you should ask specifically if he has ever had
1. Epilepsy
2. Asthma
3. Chromosome damage
*4. Porphyria

2. Your nursing assessment should include specific questions about
a. The proportion of fat included in MC's diet
b. The type of shoes MC wears
c. Skin preparations MC uses on the lower part of his body
d. Whether or not MC uses alcoholic beverages
1. a, b, c
2. a, b, d
3. a, c, d
4. b, c, d
*5. All of the above

3. MC should be informed that he will probably need periodic laboratory tests to detect changes in

a. Concentration of blood cells
b. Liver function
c. Kidney function
1. a, b
2. a, c
3. b, c
*4. All of the above

4. MC should inform the physician promptly if the following adverse reaction to griseofulvin develops:
1. Changes in visual acuity
*2. Skin rash that appears different from the tinea eruption
3. Itching in the skin area affected by the tinea eruption
4. Hypertrophy of the gums

18 Drugs Used to Treat Rickettsiae, Protozoa, Helminths, and Ectoparasites

Chapter 18 deals with drug treatment of infections and infestations caused by rickettsiae, protozoa, and macroscopic parasites such as worms and lice.

Through the study of this chapter, the student may develop the following concepts:

1 □ The most effective approach to the control of rickettsial, protozoan, and helminthic diseases is the elimination of reservoirs of infection and avoidance of exposure.
2 □ Warfarin is a rodenticide that effectively eliminates small animal vectors by impairing the coagulation process and inducing fatal hemorrhages.
3 □ Drugs used in the treatment of protozoan and systemic fungal infections have a narrow safety margin and can cause serious adverse reactions.
4 □ The choice of medication for the treatment of protozoan infection is dependent on a number of factors, including resistance of the organism, whether the disease is endemic in the area, and the general physical condition of the client.
5 □ Protozoan and helminthic infections are debilitating. Clients receiving drugs to treat these diseases require careful supportive care.
6 □ Infection by parasitic worms is found most commonly in areas with poor sanitation and living conditions.
7 □ When mixed infestations are present and more than one agent is required to treat the client, the order in which the drugs are given may be critical to prevent serious adverse reactions.
8 □ Ectoparasite infestations are highly contagious, and their incidence has risen in recent years.
9 □ Insecticides used for the treatment of ectoparasite infestations can be absorbed by the skin and may cause serious toxicity.
10 □ Ectoparasite infestations are best controlled by prevention of infestations through sanitary, hygienic, and aseptic measures.

Teaching Strategies

Students could be assigned to this chapter at the time in the curriculum when they are introduced to basic concepts of public health. Field trips to community agencies and facilities charged with maintaining sanitary facilities and waste disposal would illustrate the implementation of many of the principles of contagious disease control.

□ Topics for classroom discussions might include the following:

a. Why did the worldwide campaign to eliminate smallpox succeed, whereas the attempt to eradicate malaria did not?
b. How can nurses influence public policies related to the control of infectious diseases?
c. What are the local health ordinances pertaining to the control of insect and animal vectors involved in the transmission of contagious diseases?
d. Explore the geographic distribution of protozoan infections. Are any endemic in the local area? If so, what is done to control them? If not, are occasional cases seen in acute care institutions? How do these arise?
e. What special assessments should be made when taking a nursing history from clients who will receive antimalarial drugs? amebicides? anthelmintics?
f. Are present restrictions on the use of insecticides too stringent? too lenient? What suggestions could be made for more appropriate use of these substances?

Evaluation Examples (Test Items)

ESSAY QUESTION

A client has just moved into an old house that has been unoccupied for months. He wishes to eradicate life forms infesting the building that are apt to cause disease. He plans to fumigate and distribute poison around the home. What advice would you give him regarding initial decontamination and maintenance measures?

MULTIPLE CHOICE ITEMS

1. Active immunization against rickettsial diseases such as typhus is usually recommended
   1. Routinely at the age of 1 year
   2. Whenever a case is diagnosed in the area
   3. When the Center for Disease Control declares that an epidemic is occurring
   *4. When civil disruption or natural disaster interferes with normal sanitation measures

2. The rodenticide presently in most common use is
   1. Phosphorus
   2. Sulfur
   *3. Warfarin
   4. Strychnine

3. The drugs of choice for treating rickettsial infection are the
   1. Penicillins
   2. Aminoglycosides
   3. Erythromycins
   *4. Tetracyclines

19 Antipyretics

Fever
Pathophysiology of Fever
Defining and Diagnosing Fever
Therapeutic Management of Fever
Drugs Used to Control Fever
Nursing Management
Nursing Process
Assessment
Diagnosis
Planning
Intervention
Evaluation

Chapter 19 presents theory related to the origin of fever, its physiologic effects, and its control through the use of drugs. Drugs discussed include quinine, the glucocorticoids, dantrolene, aspirin, and acetaminophen.

Through the study of this chapter, students may develop the following concepts:

1 □ Fever has protective as well as harmful effects.
2 □ Although prolonged high fevers must be avoided, it is rarely desirable to eliminate fever completely through the use of drugs.
3 □ An optimal temperature range should be designated for clients receiving treatment intended to control fever.
4 □ Frequently used over-the-counter drugs such as aspirin have harmful effects in some clients. Use of these drugs requires as much caution as treatment with more exotic therapeutic drugs.

Teaching Strategies

The material in this chapter can be integrated effectively with content related to the measurement of vital functions (including measurement of temperature). Class discussion should draw on students' past experiences with the common antipyretic drugs aspirin and acetaminophen.

Evaluation Examples (Test Items)

ESSAY QUESTIONS

1. Describe the resolution of fever by the two processes, crisis and lysis.

2. Discuss the effects of fever on the body, both beneficial and harmful.

MULTIPLE CHOICE ITEMS

1. Fever is believed to stem *primarily* from the release by the body of
1. Calorie nutrients that are subsequently metabolized for energy
2. Thyroid hormone, which increases metabolic production of energy
*3. Polysaccharide or proteinaceous substances, which influence the hypothalamic thermostat
4. Tissue breakdown products, which act as general central nervous system stimulants

2. Body temperature is controlled *primarily* by the
1. Cerebral cortex
*2. Hypothalamus
3. Pituitary gland
4. Basal ganglia

3. Drugs employed to control fever include
a. Thyroxin
b. Epinephrine
c. Hydrocortisone
d. Morphine
e. Propoxyphene
f. Acetaminophen
g. Dantrolene
1. a, c, e, g
2. b, d, f
3. e only
4. a, b, d
*5. c, f, g

4. Dantrolene may be administered by the following routes:
1. IM, IV
2. PO, PR
3. SC, IM
*4. PO, IV

5. The herbal preparation that contains salicylate antipyretics is tea made from
*1. Willow bark
2. Cinchona bark
3. Sassafras
4. Chamomile

6. An allergic asthmatic attack is likely to develop in response to ingestion of the antipyretic drug
*1. Aspirin
2. Acetaminophen
3. Quinine
4. All of the above

7. Tinnitus is known as a side effect of the antipyretic drugs
a. Aspirin
b. Acetaminophen
c. Quinine
1. a, b

*2. a, c
3. b, c
4. All of the above

8. Body temperature is likely to be highest
1. Before a chill begins
2. During a chill, with the onset of shivering
*3. When the chill ends

SITUATION-BASED MULTIPLE CHOICE ITEMS

Situation: Mrs. FI, age 50 years, is admitted to the hospital at 11 AM with an acute respiratory tract infection. Her rectal temperature on admission is 100.8°F. A cbc, urinalysis, sputum for culture and sensitivity, chest x-ray, clear liquid diet, bed rest, and oral antibiotic have been ordered. The tests are completed, and the first dose of the antibiotic is administered by 3 PM.

1. You would anticipate that FI's temperature at 4 PM would be
1. Lower than the admission temperature
2. Approximately the same as the admission temperature
*3. Higher than the admission temperature

2. At 5 PM acetaminophen 700 mg PO or PR for rectal temperature >101°F is ordered. The maximum temperature was probably set at this level because
1. Tissue damage begins to occur when body temperature rises over 102°F.
2. At her age, FI's normal temperature is probably higher than her normal temperature when she was younger
*3. A moderate increase in temperature assists the body in resisting febrile infectious diseases
4. An error may have been made; you should verify the order

3. At 8 PM FI's temperature is 102.4°F. You would
*1. Administer the acetaminophen by mouth with a glass of water or fruit juice
2. Administer the acetaminophen by mouth with a small glass of milk
3. Administer an acetaminophen suppository by rectum to prevent gastric irritation
4. Contact the physician to verify that the antipyretic should be administered

20 Agents Used in Debridement of Wounds

Drug Agents
Anti-infectives
Hydrogen Peroxide
Proteolytic Enzymes
Absorptive Beads
Nursing Management
Nursing Implications

Chapter 20 discusses oxidizing, enzymatic, and absorptive drugs used to promote the debridement of wounds.

Through the study of this chapter, the student may develop the following concepts:

1 □ Clean wounds heal more rapidly than wounds containing tissue debris or purulent exudate.
2 □ Chemical agents supplement but do not replace mechanical methods of debridement such as irrigation, whirlpool baths, surgery, and wet-to-dry dressings.
3 □ Hydrogen peroxide solutions must be used while fresh because they break down to release oxygen and water when exposed to light and air.
4 □ Proteolytic enzymes are highly antigenic.
5 □ Proteolytic enzymes tend to promote hemorrhage because they dissolve clots.
6 □ Proteolytic enzymes must be protected from heat and agitation, which tend to denature them.
7 □ Hydrogen peroxide and dextran macromolecules cause discomfort, especially when first applied to wounds.

Teaching Strategies

This chapter on debridement could be assigned along with Chapters 15 and 17 as part of a comprehensive study of wound management. Other content appropriate to an integrated approach could include nursing skills involved in sterile asepsis, dressings, irrigations and pathophysiology related to inflammation, and localized infection.

□ Topics for classroom discussion could include the following:

a. A comparison and contrast of techniques favored by local surgeons for the debridement of wounds.

b. A comparison and contrast of client responses to various debridement regimens.

Evaluation Examples (Test Items)

ESSAY QUESTIONS

1. Compare and contrast mechanical methods of debridement with the use of drug agents for debridement, considering the following: convenience, expense, and client responses, both favorable and unfavorable.

2. Briefly describe the methods for administering two of the following drugs for the debridement of wounds: hydrogen peroxide, proteolytic enzymes, Debrisan.

SITUATION-BASED MULTIPLE CHOICE ITEMS

Situation: Ms. LD, age 63 years, has been transferred from a local nursing home to the hospital for treatment of an infected decubitus secondary to paraplegia caused by a spinal cord injury. The wound, an open crater 4" X 5" in size, is grossly infected and contains considerable necrotic material. A systemic antibiotic and hydrogen peroxide irrigations tid followed by wet-to-dry dressings have been ordered.

1. The proper concentration of hydrogen peroxide to use for wound irrigations is about
1. 1:1000 (0.1%)
*2. 1:100 (1.0%)
3. 1:10 (10%)
4. 1:1 (100%)

2. The peroxide solution should be stored in
1. The refrigerator
2. A vented container
3. A tightly closed clear bottle
*4. A tightly closed brown bottle

3. Before beginning the first irrigation, you should
1. Reassure LD that the treatment will be painless
*2. Warn LD that she may feel a stinging sensation at first
3. Medicate LD with an analgesic to prevent severe pain when the peroxide is applied

The next day, the physician discontinues the wet-to-dry dressings because their removal caused LD acute discomfort. At this time, an order is written for Elase ointment to be applied to the wound following the hydrogen peroxide irrigations.

4. Before applying the Elase ointment to the wound, you should first
1. Remove the hydrogen peroxide from the wound by sponging with a dry sterile dressing
*2. Remove the hydrogen peroxide from the wound by irrigating with normal saline solution
3. Leave a small pool of hydrogen peroxide in the

wound to prolong the antiseptic and debriding action of this solution
4. Leave a small pool of hydrogen peroxide in the wound to facilitate the action of the proteolytic medication by dissolving it

5. You should watch LD carefully for signs and symptoms of
a. Allergic reaction
b. Thrombotic emboli
c. Hemorrhage from the wound
1. a, b
*2. a, c
3. b, c
4. All of the above

21 Anti-inflammatory and Related Agents

Pathophysiology of Inflammation
The Use of Anti-inflammatory Agents
Nonsteroidal Anti-inflammatory Agents
Salicylates
Indoleacetic Acid Derivatives
Indeneacetic Acid Derivatives
Pyrrole Acetic Acid Derivatives
Propionic Acid Derivatives
Fenamic Acid Derivatives
Other Anti-inflammatory Agents
Pyrazolon Derivatives
Para-aminophenol Derivatives
Gold Compounds
Drugs Used in the Management of Gout
Colchicine
Allopurinol
Uricosurics
Probenecid
Sulfinpyrazone
Nursing Management

Chapter 21 briefly discusses the inflammatory process. Its intention is to emphasize that this process is a normal, necessary, protective mechanism for survival and that the process is not the same as infection.

Medications that have anti-inflammatory effects are discussed. Anti-infective agents are used when the inflammatory process is deleterious to the patient. Drugs in this chapter include salicylates, pyrazolon derivatives, indomethacin and sulindac, propionic acid derivatives, fenamic acid derivatives, para-aminophenol derivatives, gold, and certain drugs used to treat gout. The drugs in this group may have effects in addition to their anti-inflammatory effect, such as analgesia and antipyresis.

Through the study of this chapter, students may develop the following concepts:

1 □ Medications with anti-inflammatory effects are for use when the inflammatory process has had or would appear to be causing a deleterious effect to a client.
2 □ Most of the medications with anti-inflammatory effects probably interfere with the synthesis and release of prostaglandins in some way.
3 □ Medications with anti-inflammatory effects are usually administered orally (except gold).
4 □ Most of these medications are used for analgesia with headache, neuralgia, myalgia, dysmenorrhea, and arthralgia. With osteoarthritis and rheumatoid arthritis, joint swelling may be reduced, pain and duration of stiffness are lessened, and strength and mobility are improved.
5 □ Most of these medications share a common adverse effect—that is, disturbance of gastrointestinal system function.
6 □ Because some of these medications are so widely available without prescription, they are connected with a high incidence of toxic reactions or poisonings (*e.g.*, acetylsalicylic acid, phenacetin, acetaminophen).
7 □ Client education is crucial with use of this group of medications because of misconceptions about advertising claims, side effects, inappropriate usage by clients, and toxicity.

Teaching Strategies

1 □ Classroom discussion may be stimulated by consideration of questions such as the following:

a. What over-the-counter preparations do you and your family use that contain some of these agents? Why do you and your family use these preparations? How frequently are they used? How are they stored in the home? What improvements should be made in your home in terms of usage of these agents?
b. What advertising claims are you familiar with in relation to the over-the-counter preparations containing these agents? Examine the truth or falsity of these claims on the basis of information in the text.
c. You have a client who has used an acetylsalicylic acid preparation for years for frequent headaches. Now there is a medical indication for acetylsalicylic acid to be completely avoided. How would you help this client? What are the elements of change theory that would need to be applied?
d. Your client is being placed on long-term therapy with one of these agents for severe osteoarthritis. What questions would you ask to determine when the client should take the medication? What teaching points should be made to assist the client to avoid adverse effects?

2 □ An individual homework assignment or out-of-class group project could focus further on the over-the-counter preparations containing agents from this group of medications. Students could visit a local drugstore, obtain information from product labels about claims and contents, and study the information about contents in the text. This information could be shared in class with the other students. The information could also be typed up and placed in a looseleaf binder as a classroom "scrapbook" of information.
3 □ An out-of-class group project could focus on safety measures to take with these medications. Posters could be made and then placed in the classrooms of an elementary school as part of the health education component of the curriculum. Students highly interested in teaching and school nursing could make a short in-class presentation to the children in conjunction with the posters.

Evaluation Examples (Test Items)

MULTIPLE CHOICE ITEMS

1. The explanation for acetylsalicylic acid's anti-inflammatory action is
 1. Inhibition of phagocytosis
 2. Depression of cellular immunity
 *3. Inhibition of prostaglandin synthesis and release
 4. Reduction in capillary permeability

2. The most common adverse effect seen with acetylsalicylic acid administration is
 1. Hypersensitivity
 2. Bleeding tendency
 3. Ototoxicity
 *4. Gastrointestinal dysfunction
 5. Nephropathy

3. A drug that is *not* used routinely because of its side effects is
 1. Acetylsalicylic acid
 *2. Phenylbutazone
 3. Acetaminophen
 4. Indomethacin

4. The common trade name(s) for the preparation ibuprofen is (are)
 *1. Motrin and Rufen
 2. Naprosyn
 3. Nalfon
 4. Clinoril

5. Ibuprofen is an example of a
 1. Salicylate
 2. Para-aminophenol derivative
 3. Pyrazolon derivative
 *4. Propionic acid derivative

6. Phenacetin and acetaminophen possess the following properties:
 1. Analgesic
 *2. Analgesic, antipyretic
 3. Antipyretic, anti-inflammatory
 4. Analgesic, antipyretic, anti-inflammatory

7. Phenacetin has been implicated with the following side effect of long-term use
 1. Congestive heart failure
 *2. Analgesic abuse nephropathy
 3. Liver failure
 4. Anemia

8. The organ of the body showing the greatest toxicity with acute overdose of acetaminophen is
 1. Heart
 2. Kidney
 *3. Liver
 4. Stomach

9. An agent used in the treatment of a client with acute overdose of acetaminophen is
 1. Epinephrine
 2. Sodium bicarbonate
 *3. Acetylcysteine
 4. Fenoprofen

10. The most common side effect of gold therapy is
 1. Gastrointestinal irritation
 2. Aplastic anemia
 3. Metallic taste in mouth
 *4. Cutaneous lesions

11. Colchicine is used in the management of
 1. Ankylosing spondylitis
 *2. Gout
 3. Rheumatic fever
 4. Osteoarthritis

12. A drug that causes an increased and prolonged concentration of penicillin in the plasma is
 *1. Probenecid
 2. Indomethacin
 3. Tolmetin
 4. Acetylsalicylic acid

UNIT FIVE: DRUGS AFFECTING THE NERVOUS SYSTEM

22 Autonomic Drugs

Introduction to Drugs Affecting the Nervous System
The Autonomic Nervous System
Physiology of the Autonomic Nervous System
Adrenergic Compounds
Catecholamines
Noncatecholamines
Nursing Management
Adrenergic Blocking Agents
Alpha-adrenergic Blocking Agents
Beta-adrenergic Blocking Agents
Adrenergic Neuron Blocking Agents
Nursing Management
Cholinergic Drugs
Parasympathomimetic Agents
Anticholinesterase Agents
Nursing Management
Anticholinergic Drugs
Atropine
Scopolamine and Synthetic and Semisynthetic Antimuscarinics
Nursing Management
Ganglionic Stimulants
Nicotine
Ganglionic Blocking Agents

Six classes of drugs are discussed in Chapter 22. Included in this group is a major drug of abuse that produces both physical and psychologic dependence: nicotine.

Through study of this chapter, the student may develop the following concepts:

1 □ Autonomic drugs may be very general in their action, interacting with all types of receptors in a division of the system (sympathetic or parasympathetic), or they may be somewhat selective, interacting only with specific subtypes of receptors such as ß-adrenergic receptors.

2 □ The more selective the action of a drug, the fewer adverse reactions caused by it.

3 □ Continuous intravenous infusions of potent drugs should be controlled by mechanical regulators or infusion pumps.

4 □ Mechanical regulators must be monitored to ensure safety in drug administration.

5 □ Drug interactions may be both beneficial (*e.g.*, epinephrine, local anesthetics) or harmful (*e.g.*, epinephrine, halogenated hydrocarbon anesthetics).

6 □ Adrenergic decongestants act as vasopressors and central nervous system stimulants.

7 □ Adrenergic decongestants may cause dependence as a result of rebound vasodilation.

8 □ Epinephrine is the drug of choice for initial treatment of anaphylactic shock.

9 □ Amphetamines have limited medical uses. They are recommended for the treatment of narcolepsy, parkinsonism, minimal brain damage syndrome, and absence seizures. They are not recommended for the treatment of obesity.

10 □ Drugs influencing the autonomic nervous system can influence emotional affect and mood.

11 □ ß-Adrenergic blocking agents protect the heart from tachycardia and hypertension caused by sympathetic stimulation.

12 □ Antidotes for autonomic drugs are drugs that exert opposite effects on the autonomic nervous system (*e.g.*, phentolamine is the antidote for norepinephrine, while atropine antagonizes the effects of cholinergic drugs).

13 □ Cholinergic drugs increase the likelihood of allergic reaction and may precipitate allergic reactions in susceptible persons.

14 □ Cholinergic excess produces muscular weakness that resembles cholinergic deficiency.

15 □ Interruption of drug therapy or a drop in serum drug concentrations in myasthenia gravis can cause respiratory paralysis and death.

16 □ Anticholinergic drugs may cause acute glaucoma and acute urinary retention in susceptible clients. They also affect potency in men adversely.

17 □ Drugs administered topically to the mucous membranes can cause toxic symptoms because of absorption into the systemic circulation.

18 □ Nicotine affects the central nervous system as well as the autonomic system. Its action is biphasic—first stimulation, followed by depression.

19 □ Nicotine is a potent vasoconstrictor; it causes physical and psychologic dependence. Cigarette smoking increases the risk of serious diseases such as peptic ulcer, obstructive airway disease, cardiovascular disease, cancer, and complications of pregnancy.

20 □ As a group, autonomic drugs tend to be potent; dosages are often measured in micrograms.

Teaching Strategies

1 □ The study of autonomic drugs is an appropriate opportunity to discuss both the use of drugs to support vital functions during emergencies and the problem of drug dependence. Epinephrine and atropine are among the most frequently used agents to combat life-threatening conditions such as anaphylaxis or acute allergic asthma. If students are involved in clinical laboratory

experiences, they should examine emergency drug supplies and become familiar with the location and type of drugs kept readily available in institutions for emergency use. They should also study the policies and procedures developed by institutions to ensure that proper action will be taken to treat acutely ill clients in need of emergency care.

2 □ Classroom discussion could consider the following:

a. What measures are taken to ensure that emergency drugs are readily available when needed?

b. What routes of administration are used for delivering drug doses when rapid effect is required?

c. How is staff function organized to minimize confusion and wasted effort during emergency treatment?

d. How are emergency drugs secured when not in use?

3 □ This chapter introduces two drugs involved in abuse by a significant number of people: amphetamines and nicotine. Nicotine is legal, readily available, and socially acceptable, whereas amphetamines are limited to prescription use, use for psychoactive effect is illegal, and abuse is not socially acceptable. It is believed that nicotine is used by greater numbers of people than amphetamines, although this is difficult to verify because amphetamine abuse is illegal and tends to be hidden.

Classroom discussion about drug abuse might consider the following questions:

a. What environmental factors influence people toward the use of drugs for psychoactive effects?

b. What are the risk factors predisposing a person to inappropriate drug use?

c. How do cultural traditions influence the use of psychoactive drugs?

d. What approaches have proven most effective in assisting people to overcome dependence on drugs?

Evaluation Examples (Test Items)

ESSAY QUESTIONS

1. Outline a teaching plan for a lesson on the use and abuse of stimulant drugs for an elementary school class.

2. Describe the "flight-fright-fight" reaction characteristic of adrenergic stimulation. Which of the signs and symptoms are caused by epinephrine secretion and which are norepinephrine secretion?

3. Describe both phases of nicotine's effects on the body. Which of these effects contribute to the development of disease?

4. Describe two mechanisms of action whereby autonomic drugs function. Give examples of drugs that act by each mechanism.

5. Select *one* of the following drugs and briefly describe its place in drug therapy: epinephrine, atropine, neostigmine, propanolol. Include the following: the class(es) or family(ies) of drugs to which the drug belongs; its mechanisms of action, therapeutic uses, common side effects, toxic effects, and potential for idiosyncratic or allergic reaction; and antidotes or recommended treatment for toxicity.

6. Compare and contrast the mechanisms of action of atropine and epinephrine.

MULTIPLE CHOICE ITEMS

1. Adrenergic drugs are substances that produce a physiologic response resembling that of
1. Parasympathetic stimulation
2. Parasympathetic inhibition
*3. Sympathetic stimulation
4. Sympathetic inhibition

2. Adrenergic drugs tend to cause the following side effects
a. Vasodilation
b. Central nervous system stimulation
c. Muscle tremor
1. a, b
2. a, c
*3. b, c
4. All of the above

3. The drug of choice for treatment of anaphylaxis is
1. Atropine
2. Neostigmine
3. Propanolol
*4. Epinephrine

4. Epinephrine is usually administered
1. Orally
2. By inhalation
*3. By injection
4. Transdermally

5. Propranolol exerts its pharmacologic actions by
1. Stimulating ß-adrenergic receptors
*2. Blocking ß-adrenergic receptors
3. Stimulating cholinergic receptors
4. Blocking cholinergic receptors

SITUATION-BASED MULTIPLE CHOICE ITEMS

Situation: Your client, Ms. AO, is a 20-year-old college student who fell into a coma following ingestion of an unknown quantity of "reds" (secobarbital capsules). To support vital functions, she is mechanically ventilated by an endotracheal tube and is receiving continuous intravenous norepinephrine to maintain blood pressure.

1. You should take the blood pressure every
1. 15 to 30 minutes if outside the parameters selected by the physician
2. 15 to 30 minutes if the dosage of norepinephrine has been altered

*3. 2 to 5 minutes until both the dosage of norepinephrine and blood pressure have been stabilized
4. 2 to 5 minutes until AO regains consciousness

2. You should be most careful to observe her for
1. Cardiac arrhythmias
2. Infection at the site of the IV
*3. Infiltration of the IV
4. Bronchospasm

3. What is the antidote for norepinephrine?
*1. Phentolamine
2. Propranolol
3. Epinephrine
4. Atropine

4. You discover infiltration of the tissues around the site of the IV line carrying the norepinephrine. What should be done?
1. The intravenous infusion should be speeded up
2. A dose of the antidote should be administered through the IV line
3. A dose of the antidote should be administered by nebulization through the endotracheal tube
*4. A dose of the antidote should be injected directly into the tissues around the IV site

Situation: You are working in the emergency room when 14-year-old TH is admitted in acute respiratory distress manifested by tachypnea and wheezing. He appears frightened. A diagnosis of acute asthma is made, and TH is given 0.3 ml of 1:1000 epinephrine.

1. The dosage of drug TH received is equivalent to
1. 0.03 mg (30 μg)
*2. 0.3 mg (300 μg)
3. 3 mg
4. 30 mg (0.03 g)

2. TH's respirations decrease and become quiet. However, he continues to appear apprehensive and restless. You should tell him that these feelings are
a. Caused in part by a change in the acid-base balance that has resulted from hyperventilation
b. Caused in part by effects of the drug on the central nervous system
c. Temporary in nature and will decrease as the drug wears off
1. a, b
2. a, c
*3. b, c
4. All of the above

3. TH is admitted for observation and continued treatment. He is likely to continue to receive adrenergic drugs to control bronchospasm. An important nursing intervention during this period is
1. Assisting TH to control calorie intake to prevent weight gain
2. Observing TH for respiratory alkalosis secondary to hyperventilation induced by the medications
3. Frequent mouth care to alleviate dry mouth caused by the drugs
*4. Measures to promote rest and sleep

Situation: One of the residents in the nursing home in which you work, Ms. MY, has recently been diagnosed as having myasthenia gravis, for which neostigmine has been prescribed. Medication is scheduled to be given before each meal, at bedtime, and at 2 AM.

1. MY's daughter asks you why her mother is being awakened in the middle of the night for medication. You tell her that
1. The drug is administered to promote adequate REM sleep
2. The night dose may not be necessary once MY adjusts to the medication
*3. The night dose is essential to maintain normal respirations
4. Both 1 and 2 above

2. MY responds well to the medication during the first week of treatment. On the tenth day of the regimen, she again experiences difficulty in breathing and complains of renewed weakness. A review of her chart verifies that the medication has been administered consistently, as ordered. MY's symptoms are probably a result of
1. An acute respiratory infection
2. A rapidly developing resistance to the effects of the medication
3. Rapid progression of the underlying disease
*4. Accumulation of the medication, causing cholinergic crisis

3. Appropriate nursing actions in the above situation include contacting the physician and
a. Requesting an antibiotic order
b. Requesting an order for increasing the dosage of neostigmine
c. Delaying the next dose of neostigmine
d. Preparing for respiratory resuscitation
1. a only
2. b, d
*3. c, d
4. a, c
5. b only

4. A drug that is generally contraindicated by MY would be
*1. Atropine
2. Edrophonium
3. Epinephrine
4. Propranolol

23
Central Nervous System Stimulants

Physiology of the Central Nervous System
Central Nervous System Stimulants
Amphetamines
Xanthines
Levodopa
Analeptics
Cocaine
Khat and Betel
Hallucinogens

Chapter 23 introduces central nervous system (CNS) drugs with a brief review of CNS structure and function, and a discussion of CNS stimulants. Both beneficial and harmful effects of the drugs are included in order to promote the concept that chemicals are not intrinsically good or bad but have the potential for both benefit and harm.

Through the study of this chapter, the student may develop the following concepts:

1 □ Chemical substances are neither good nor bad but have the potential for both benefit and harm, depending on the way they are used.
2 □ Chemicals that influence nervous system function have wide-ranging effects on physical functions, emotional states, and mental capacity.
3 □ Distribution of drugs within the CNS is controlled by the blood-brain barrier.
4 □ Response to CNS drugs is influenced by characteristics of the client such as physiologic function, emotional mood, and mental set.
5 □ Exposure to CNS drugs tends to produce tolerance; many of these drugs cause psychologic or physical dependence.
6 □ In most cultures, the chronic use of one or more CNS drugs is accepted social practice.
7 □ Chemical changes are believed to underly many physical and mental illnesses characterized by altered brain function.
8 □ Although current knowledge about CNS function and the pharmacodynamics of CNS drugs is too inadequate to provide a rational basis for treatment, it is likely that drug therapy has the potential for correcting abnormal brain chemistry, thereby controlling or curing illness caused by brain malfunction.
9 □ CNS stimulants increase mental alertness and capacity for work. Large doses cause tremor, insomnia, hallucinations, and convulsions. Prolonged use leads to exhaustion.
10 □ Accurate assessment of the potential of CNS drugs to produce dependency requires years of experience in use of the drugs.

Teaching Strategies

The treatment accorded CNS drugs may heavily influence student attitudes toward drug use in general. The substances discussed in this chapter and Chapter 24 are among the most frequently used therapeutic agents and the most frequently abused street drugs. If a balanced approach based on rational evaluation without emotional or ethical overtones can be maintained, student biases regarding drugs may be reduced considerably. It is recommended that each drug be discussed holistically, with consideration of its potential for both therapeutic benefit and detrimental effects.

1 □ Students should be encouraged to explore their own attitudes toward drug use and the experiences that shaped them. Clinical examples can illustrate the influence of nurses' attitudes on therapeutic uses of drugs. A knowledge and understanding of personal bias is necessary if its influence on behavior is to be minimized by compensatory adaptations. If instructors share their own biases relating to drugs and the corrective measures used to prevent these biases from influencing clinical judgment, a role model will be provided for students to follow.
2 □ Classroom discussion might consider the following questions:

a. What factors influence the development of attitudes toward drug use?
b. What are the common effects of large doses of CNS stimulants?
c. What emergency treatment is required for people who have taken overdoses of CNS stimulants?
d. What CNS stimulants are used most frequently in the local health-care settings? In the community?
e. What community resources are available for the treatment of clients with drug dependence? Is a stigma attached to use of these facilities?

3 □ Chapter 48 deals with substance abuse and may be integrated into this chapter.

Evaluation Examples (Test Items)

ESSAY QUESTION

1. Describe what you believe to be your personal biases toward the use of drugs. If you are aware of experiences that influenced your attitude, indicate their nature. How do you think these feelings might influence your nursing care of clients taking drugs?

SITUATION-BASED MULTIPLE CHOICE ITEMS

Situation: AS, 8 years old, has been brought to the pediatrician for evaluation because of episodic temper tantrums and inconsistent scholastic performance related to a short attention span. The physician believes that AS has minimal brain dysfunction (MBD) and prescribes an amphetamine preparation for her to take daily when school is in session.

1. While you are explaining the treatment plan to AS's mother, she expresses dismay over giving Alice "addictive" drugs. Your best response would be that

1. Amphetamines do not cause dependence and are not considered to be addictive
2. Physical dependence on amphetamines is treatable by gradual reduction in dosage
3. Psychologic dependence on amphetamines can sometimes become a problem, but the benefits of taking the drug outweigh the risk of dependence

*4. The degree to which amphetamines cause dependence is uncertain, but children who have taken these drugs for MBD do not appear to develop dependence

2. When should AS receive her daily medication?

*1. After arising in the morning
2. At lunchtime
3. After school
4. At bedtime

3. AS's mother asks you, "Should I omit the medication on weekends, or just during vacations?" Your best response would be

1. Continue the medication over school recesses of less than 1 week, but discontinue it for vacations of a week or more
2. Give the medication only on days AS attends school

*3. Give the medication on days when AS is called on to perform intellectually, whether it is at school or in some other learning situation
4. Give the medication regularly until AS's symptoms subside, and then reduce the dosage to the minimally effective level

4. AS asks you, "How long will I have to take the medicine?" Your best reply would be

1. You will probably need to take the medicine indefinitely

*2. You will probably outgrow your need for the medicine eventually
3. You will probably be taking the medicine for a year or two
4. After a few weeks of medication, you will probably be able to take it on a PRN basis

5. To prepare AS and her mother to cope with side effects of the medication, you should

a. Demonstrate techniques of massage to relieve stiff muscles
b. Teach measures to promote rest and sleep
c. Recommend that AS drink a cup of coffee when she takes her medication

*1. a, b
2. a, c
3. b, c
4. All of the above

24 Central Nervous System Depressants

Anesthetics
- *General Anesthetics*
- *Local Anesthetics*
- *Alternative Anesthetic Regimens*

Analgesics
- *Opiates and Opioids*
- *Nonnarcotic Opioid Receptor Agonists*
- *Opioid Antagonists*

Hypnotics
- *Physiology of Sleep*
- *Stages and Patterns of Sleep*
- *Pathophysiology of Sleep Disorders*
- *Hypnotic Drugs*

Alcohol
- *Ethyl Alcohol*
- *Toxic Alcohols*
- *Disulfiram Therapy*

Chapter 24 discusses central nervous system (CNS) depressants, a group of substances widely used both in medical therapy and for psychoactive effects. Some of the oldest drugs used to relieve pain are included in this group. Therapeutic agents discussed in detail include anesthetics, analgesics, and sedative–hypnotics. Drugs of abuse included in this chapter include opiates, barbiturates, and alcohol. Both beneficial and harmful aspects of each drug are discussed to promote the concept that chemicals are not in themselves good or bad but have potential for both benefit and harm.

Through the study of this chapter, the student may develop the following concepts:

1 □ Chemical substances are neither good nor bad but have the potential for both benefit and harm, depending on the way they are used.
2 □ Chemicals that influence nervous system function have wide-ranging effects on physical functions, emotional states, and mental capacity.
3 □ Distribution of drugs within the CNS is controlled by the blood-brain barrier.
4 □ Response to CNS drugs is influenced by characteristics of the client such as physiologic function, emotional mood, and mental set.
5 □ Exposure to CNS drugs tends to produce tolerance; many of these drugs cause psychologic or physical dependence.
6 □ In most cultures, the chronic use of one or more CNS drugs is accepted social practice.
7 □ Chemical changes are believed to underly many physical and mental illnesses characterized by altered brain function.
8 □ Initial effects of CNS depressants may be stimulant in nature because of depression of inhibitory functions of the brain; large doses cause stupor and coma.
9 □ Special preparation and training are required for safe administration of general anesthesia.
10 □ Responses to placebos involve real physiologic changes in body function.
11 □ Accurate assessment of the potential of CNS drugs to produce dependency requires years of experience in use of the drugs.
12 □ Chronic use of hypnotics is undesirable because all hypnotic drugs appear to disturb normal sleep stages to some degree.
13 □ Parenting practices that foster strong self-images and self-confidence in children help to reduce the risk of serious substance abuse.
14 □ Psychological dependence on drugs is more difficult to resolve than physical dependence.
15 □ Peer group support is an effective approach to control of drug dependence.

Teaching Strategies

The treatment accorded CNS drugs may heavily influence student attitudes toward drug use in general. The substances discussed in this chapter and Chapter 23 are among the most frequently used therapeutic agents and the most frequently abused street drugs. If a balanced approach based on rational evaluation without emotional or ethical overtones can be maintained, student biases regarding drugs may be reduced considerably. It is recommended that each drug be discussed holistically, with consideration of its potential for both therapeutic benefit and detrimental effects.

1 □ Students should be encouraged to explore their own attitudes toward drug use and the experiences that shaped them. Clinical examples can illustrate the influence of nurses' attitudes on therapeutic uses of drugs. A knowledge and understanding of personal bias is necessary if its influence on behavior is to be minimized by compensatory adaptations. If instructors share their own biases relating to drugs and the corrective measures used to prevent these biases from influencing clinical judgment, a role model will be provided for students to follow.
2 □ The study of anesthetics and analgesics can appropriately be integrated with theoretic material related to surgery and the operative experience. Consideration of sedative–hypnotics promotes learning most effectively when students begin evening clinical experience in institutional settings, because at this time they are actively involved in promoting sleep for their clients.

3 □ Classroom discussion might consider the following questions:

a. What factors influence the development of attitudes toward drug use?

b. How do the personal biases of the nurse influence the therapeutic administration of CNS drugs?

c. What are the common effects of large doses of CNS depressants?

d. What emergency treatment is required for people who have received overdoses of CNS depressants?

e. What CNS depressants are used most frequently in local health-care settings? In the community?

f. How does nursing practice influence the administration of drugs ordered PRN?

g. What are the prevailing biases among local nurses in relation to CNS drugs?

h. What community resources are available for the treatment of clients with drug dependence? Is a stigma attached to use of these facilities?

4 □ Chapter 48 deals with substance abuse and may be integrated into this chapter.

Evaluation Examples (Test Items)

ESSAY QUESTIONS

1. Describe what you believe to be your personal biases toward the use of drugs. If you are aware of experiences that influenced your attitude, indicate their nature. How do you think these feelings might influence your nursing care of clients taking drugs?

2. Discuss the mechanisms of action of opiates and opiate antagonists (*i.e.*, narcotic antagonists) on the nervous system.

MULTIPLE CHOICE ITEMS

1. Select the answer that best describes statements a and b.

a. In the treatment of heroin addiction, physical dependence is more difficult to eliminate than psychologic dependence.
b. The treatment of heroin addiction usually requires many months.

1. Both a and b are true, and a helps to explain b
2. Both a and b are true, but a does not help to explain b
*3. a is false and b is true
4. Both a and b are false

2. You have prepared the first dose of aspirin and diazepam (Valium) to administer to a newly admitted client. The client looks at the pills and asks, "Is that Valium? I can't take Valium." Your best reply would be

1. "We are not allowed to tell you what drugs have been ordered for you."
2. "You may have had difficulty with Valium before, but here in the hospital it is safer to take because you are observed closely and can be treated quickly."
3. "I'll call the physician and ask for a change in the drug order."
*4. "What happens when you take Valium?"

SITUATION-BASED MULTIPLE CHOICE ITEMS

Situation: Ms. HR, 54 years old, has terminal metastatic cancer of the breast. She is extremely debilitated and unable to ambulate. To control pain, she is receiving morphine by continuous intravenous infusion. This morning, HR inadvertently received an overdose of morphine equivalent to 200 mg. She has become stuporous and is breathing at the rate of six per minute.

1. Your *first* action should be to

1. Attempt to stimulate HR verbally to breathe faster
2. Remove the intravenous line
*3. Stop the morphine infusion, keeping the intravenous line open with a drug-free solution
4. Maintain the intravenous infusion but inject enough opioid antagonist to neutralize the 200 mg of morphine

2. If HR stops breathing, what should you do?

1. Increase the dose of morphine antagonist given intravenously
*2. Call the resuscitation team and start mouth-to-mouth breathing
3. Notify the physician that HR has apparently expired

3. What drug is most likely to be used as an antagonist for morphine?

1. Picrotoxin
2. Nalorphine
3. Pentazocine
*4. Naloxone

4. Optimum dosage of morphine antagonist for HR would be

1. Sufficient to restore respirations to normal but not enough to restore consciousness
*2. Sufficient to restore respirations and consciousness but not enough to abolish all morphine effect
3. Sufficient to abolish all the effects of morphine
4. None of the above; an antidote is not indicated for this client because of her terminal state

5. When a morphine antagonist is employed, you would anticipate that the drug be administered

1. Once only in sufficient dosage to neutralize the morphine present in the client's system
2. Once daily until the residual opioid effects are considered to be nonthreatening to the client
*3. Repeatedly at frequent intervals to maintain blockade of the opioid receptor until most of the morphine has been eliminated from the body

4. Periodically for at least a week, because morphine is eliminated slowly from the body

6. Adverse reactions to morphine antagonists include
   a. Precipitation of an opioid withdrawal syndrome
   b. Cardiovascular collapse
   c. Recurrence of severe pain
   1. a, b
   *2. a, c
   3. b, c
   4. All of the above

25 Anticonvulsants

Pathophysiology of Seizures
Factors Affecting Occurrence of Seizures
Treatment with Drugs
Hydantoins
Barbiturates
Oxazolidinediones
Succinimides
Carbamazepine
Valproate
Benzodiazepines
Miscellaneous Agents
Calcium Channel Blockers
Nursing Management
Nursing Implications
Nursing Process

Chapter 25 focuses on seizure disorders and their management. Seizures and factors affecting the occurrence of seizures are discussed prior to a discussion of drugs used in convulsive disorders. Nursing management includes measures to reduce incidence of seizures and treatment of status epilepticus.

Through the study of this chapter, the student may develop the following concepts:

1 □ The seizure threshold varies from person to person and from time to time in any one person.
2 □ Seizure activity may occur spontaneously or in response to environmental stimuli.
3 □ Anticonvulsant drugs act to reduce impulse discharge from initiating foci or to inhibit the spread of impulses in the brain.
4 □ Seizure activity involves various physiologic phenomena; consciousness is not always lost.
5 □ Two or more anticonvulsant drugs are often required to control seizure disorders.
6 □ Most anticonvulsant drugs are central nervous system depressants; decreased mental alertness and difficulty in performing intellectual work are frequent troublesome side effects.
7 □ Brain damage can cause seizures; conversely, seizures can cause brain damage.
8 □ Most anticonvulsants are teratogenic; dosages should be reduced to a minimum before women with seizure disorders attempt to conceive.
9 □ Medication administered for prevention of seizures is usually administered orally. Treatment of status epilepticus requires administration by injection.
10 □ Control of seizure disorders can be enhanced through good hygiene and manipulation of environmental factors favoring seizure activity.

Teaching Strategies

□ The impact of seizure disorders on the life of clients can be graphically illustrated through exposure to an articulate person who is receiving drugs for the control of seizures. Students learning about anticonvulsant therapy are enriched by the use of clients as guest speakers, or as members of a panel. People exhibiting various types of seizures should be included. The discussion might explore the emotional impact of the diagnosis of seizure disorders, stigmatizing of the epileptic, factors known to precipitate seizures, measures taken (in addition to medication) to prevent seizures, the drug regimen prescribed, problems related to the maintenance of the drug regimen, and adverse reactions to the medications.

Evaluation Examples (Test Items)

ESSAY QUESTIONS

1. Briefly describe the pathophysiology underlying the phenomenon of seizures. Indicate the nature of the tissue changes found in the brain, the sequence of events that precede a seizure, and the factors operating in the spontaneous termination of seizures. Indicate what mechanisms of action are involved when diazepam is used to treat acute status epilepticus.

2. Briefly describe the pharmacodynamics, therapeutic uses of, and adverse reactions caused by *one* of the following anticonvulsant drugs: phenytoin, phenobarbital, trimethadione, or ethosuximide.

SITUATION-BASED MULTIPLE CHOICE ITEMS

Situation: At 6 years of age, Ms. MS is placed on ethosuximide medication to control absence seizures (petit mal epilepsy). While receiving this drug, she is to be monitored regularly by blood tests.

1. You would explain to MS and her mother that the full effect of the medication will be experienced
1. Within 1 to 2 days
*2. Within a week
3. Within a month
4. Only if relatively large doses are taken for the first 2 days

2. MS's mother asks why the blood tests are required. Your best reply would be
1. Serum drug concentrations must be monitored to prevent toxic reaction
2. Complete blood counts are needed to detect excessive concentrations of blood cells that sometimes occur
*3. Complete blood counts are needed to detect diminished blood cell concentrations that sometimes occur
4. Liver and kidney function must be monitored while ethosuximide is used

3. Her mother states that MS's "spells" occur most often when she is ill or when her usual routine is disrupted, and asks, "Can she omit the drugs when things are going all right?" You should reply that

a. Prevention of seizures is important, and the drug should be taken regularly
b. Omitting one dose probably will have no effect on MS
c. Abrupt discontinuation of the drug may cause onset of a prolonged seizure (petit mal status)
d. Once the seizures are under control, the dose may be tapered down to a minimally effective level

1. a only
*2. a, c
3. b, d
4. c only

4. MS asks, "Will I always have to take medicine?" Your best reply would be that

1. She will probably need to take some kind of medicine from now on
*2. She may outgrow the need for medicine
3. Once the seizures have been controlled for a year, the medicine will probably be withdrawn gradually on a trial basis
4. Once the seizures subside, the medicine can be taken on a PRN basis

Situation: A few days after fall term started, Mr. TW visited the college infirmary with complaints of being unable to study because of drowsiness and lethargy. His general health is good, but he had been taking phenobarbital and phenytoin for a grand mal seizure disorder. During the past spring semester TW experienced two seizures, and the dosage of his medications were increased. He has had no seizures since then, but complains that the summer was a "bummer" because he felt "dull."

1. It is most likely that the physician will

1. Substitute an anticonvulsant drug that does not cause marked sedation for the phenytoin
2. Decrease the drug dosages to the levels that TW took before last spring
*3. Gradually decrease dosages of the drugs while monitoring TW closely
4. Discontinue medication to see whether TW has outgrown his need for medication

2. To assist TW to control his seizure disorder better, you should first

*1. Assess TW's self-care habits while living independently on campus
2. Suggest that TW consider dropping some activities and "take it easy"
3. Recommend that TW engage in vigorous activity such as cross-country jogging every day

3. TW tells you that he is a "night owl" and likes to sleep late. He eats a well-balanced diet but sometimes skips breakfast. He likes ballroom dancing. Which of these practices tends to increase the likelihood of seizure?

1. Sleeping late, because it delays the time at which he takes his medication
*2. Missing meals, because his blood sugar level tends to drop
3. His diet, because the normal diet tends to cause metabolic acidosis

4. TW also says that he sometimes pulls an "all-nighter" (stays up all night). He is taking swimming lessons and avoids high-calorie foods so as to lose weight. He has been losing about 1 pound a week since returning to school. What further advice would you give him?

*1. Staying up all night increases the risk of seizure because of hormonal changes associated with exhaustion
2. Swimming may be harmful because blood oxygen levels tend to decrease
3. Losing weight causes an acid-base imbalance that can increase the risk of seizures
4. None of the above activities are likely to affect the seizure disorder

Situation: Mrs. SG, married 1 year, consults you because she and her husband would like to start a family. She has had a seizure disorder since childhood and is still taking anticonvulsant medications.

1. SG asks you if epilepsy will affect her ability to have children. Appropriate responses include the following:

a. You should ask your physician to reduce the drug dosage as much as possible before you become pregnant
b. You need to maintain good control of the seizure disorder because seizures can be harmful to the fetus
c. It is likely that one or more of your children will have some type of congenital abnormality if you continue to take drugs during pregnancy

*1. a, b
2. a, c
3. b, c
4. All of the above

2. The dosages of anticonvulsants are reduced, but the drugs cannot be discontinued. Six months later, SG learns that she is pregnant. She asks you why taking anticonvulsant drugs is undesirable during pregnancy. The most appropriate response is that anticonvulsant drugs increase the risk of

1. Spontaneous abortion
*2. Congenital defects in the baby
3. Toxemia of pregnancy
4. Depressed respirations in the newborn

3. SG is considering breast-feeding her infant. You should tell her that

1. Generally, anticonvulsant drugs are not distributed in milk
*2. Although many anticonvulsants are distributed in milk, the effect on the infant varies from drug to drug
3. It is advisable to breast-feed only if the anticonvulsant drug can be discontinued
4. Mothers with seizure disorders should not breast-feed

26
The Psychoactive Drugs

In Chapter 26 the student is helped to understand the use of drugs in treating the mentally and emotionally disturbed client. Categories of psychoactive drugs are defined and discussed, and the action of these drugs on the nervous system and their influence on client behavior is identified. The student is helped to relate the type of antipsychotic agent to the specific behavior requiring drug therapy.

The section on antipsychotic agents discusses phenothiazines in detail; the other classes of antipsychotic drugs are discussed only as they differ from the phenothiazines. Antidepressants–mood stabilizers, antianxiety agents, and anticholinergics (used to treat drug-induced parkinsonism) are discussed in a similar manner. The student is further helped to understand the most commonly diagnosed illness, depression, its underlying factors, and its most common symptoms.

The section on nursing actions discusses those interventions taken generally for all psychoactive drugs, as well as those interventions specific to each category: antipsychotics, anxiolytics, antimanics, antidepressants, and antiparkinsonism agents.

By studying this chapter, students may develop the following concepts:

1 □ Specific types of drugs are used to modify specific behaviors.
2 □ Each of the psychoactive drugs has a specific behavior modification purpose.
3 □ The nurse has specific roles and functions when administering drugs, and the implications for nursing care are specifically defined.

Teaching Strategies

1 □ For classroom discussion, have students discuss client situations in which the client receives an antipsychotic, antianxiety, antidepressant, or antimanic agent. Identify specific behavior indicating drug use, the observed effect on client behavior, the drug dosage as compared to the usual dosage, and contraindications. Compare the antipsychotic agents with the antianxiety agents.
2 □ Small groups of students may play roles. Have students play clients receiving a phenothiazine, benzodiazepine, or tricyclic antidepressant. Have them discuss their feelings involved in knowing they are receiving a psychoactive agent. How much stigma is involved? Would they want a classmate, friend, or their instructor to know that they are receiving such a medication? How would they feel if they were admitted to a mental health unit? What would be their major fears or concerns when on such medication?
3 □ In small groups, students may design a care plan for a client exhibiting psychotic behavior and receiving a phenothiazine. Do the same for a client receiving MAO inhibitors and for a client on lithium.
4 □ Discuss the reasons for the high rate of noncompliance in clients on psychoactive medications.
5 □ Identify each area that should be included when teaching a client or family about lithium. Design a teaching–learning plan for a selected drug.
6 □ Compare the tricyclic and heterocyclics to the MAO inhibitors.
7 □ Using a client situation, present data, have students formulate a nursing diagnosis, and identify appropriate interventions.

Evaluation Examples (Test Items)

MULTIPLE CHOICE ITEMS

1. In modifying psychotic symptoms, the phenothiazines appear to inhibit the subcortical areas of the brain. This includes all *but* the
1. Hypothalamus
2. Limbic system
*3. Pons

4. Reticular activating system

2. A client is admitted to the unit with auditory hallucinations and distorted thought processes. The drug of choice would most likely be

1. Diazepam
*2. Phenothiazine
3. Imipramine
4. Tricyclic agent

3. One of the most commonly occurring side effects of the phenothiazines is orthostatic hypotension. An appropriate nursing intervention would be to

1. Reduce the dosage to a more tolerated level
2. Refuse to administer the drug
*3. Encourage the client to lie down for an hour
4. Contact the physician for an order for an antiparkinsonism agent

4. Artane, 1 mg, has been ordered to be given immediately. The nurse might expect the client to have

1. Auditory hallucinations
2. Severe anxiety with agitation
3. Hypomania
*4. Extrapyramidal symptoms

UNIT SIX: DRUGS AFFECTING THE CARDIOVASCULAR SYSTEM

27 Cardiac Drugs

Physiology of the Heart
Chemical Effects on the Heart
Cardiotonics
The Cardiac Glycosides
Nursing Management in Acute Heart Failure
Nursing Management of Chronic Cardiac Conditions
Nursing Management of Acute Toxicity from Cardiac Glycosides
Antiarrhythmics
Pathophysiology of Abnormal Cardiac Rhythms
Treatment of Cardiac Arrhythmias
Antiarrhythmic Drugs
Nursing Management

Chapter 27 reviews the physiology of the heart as a basis for the student's understanding of Chapters 28 and 29. Drugs administered for their direct effect on the heart, cardiotonics and antiarrhythmics, are discussed along with management of acute and chronic congestive heart failure and arrhythmias.

Through the study of this chapter, the student may develop the following concepts:

1 □ Drugs may produce positive or negative chronotropic, dromotropic, or inotropic effects on the heart.
2 □ The action of drugs may be critically influenced by electrolyte levels; changes in electrolyte concentrations may increase the toxicity or decrease the therapeutic effects of drugs.
3 □ Toxic signs and symptoms occur more readily when drug preparations have a narrow margin of safety.
4 □ The signs and symptoms of drug toxicity sometimes mimic the signs and symptoms of the disease for which they are prescribed.
5 □ Administration of drugs must be suspended when toxic signs and symptoms occur; when a drug with a narrow safety margin is given, clients must be evaluated for early toxicity before each dose.
6 □ Cardiac drugs may be administered over long periods of time to control chronic heart disease.
7 □ Loading doses of drugs may be many times larger than maintenance doses.
8 □ Drugs that influence impulse conduction in the heart can both correct and induce cardiac arrhythmias.
9 □ Antiarrhythmic drugs influence automaticity, excitability, and conductivity of heart muscle, as well as the rate of heart contraction.
10 □ Cardioversion is the conversion of atrial fibrillation to normal rhythm. Cardioversion may be accomplished by physical means (electroshock defibrillation) or chemical means (antiarrhythmic drugs).
11 □ Thrombi in the atria formed during fibrillation are likely to dislodge and form arterial emboli when cardioversion occurs.
12 □ The treatment of heart disease often involves the use of multiple drugs (*e.g.,* cardiotonics, antiarrhythmics, and anticoagulants) as well as altered diet.
13 □ The side effects of drugs used to treat one disease may be exploited for the treatment of very different conditions.
14 □ Additives in medicinal preparations may have harmful effects on some recipients.
15 □ When a drug used for long-term therapy is initiated, close observation for adverse reactions must be maintained; monitoring sometimes requires hospitalization until the client has been stabilized on a maintenance dose.

Teaching Strategies

The study of drug therapy of cardiovascular disease is fairly complex. Multiple drugs are usually involved and interactions among drugs and between drugs and foods are frequent. If students are introduced to the study of these drugs before (or very early in) the clinical phase of their nursing education, content is best limited to pharmacodynamics and the relation of these to cardiovascular physiology. Detailed discussion of cardiovascular drugs is best delayed until a comprehensive study of cardiovascular disease is undertaken. At that time, Chapters 28, 29, and 38 could be studied together along with the pathophysiology, medical treatment, and nursing care of clients with these conditions.

1 □ Classroom discussion could consider such questions as:

a. What observations should be made when assessing clients receiving digitalis for therapeutic response? for toxicity?
b. How is cardiac response to digitalis influenced by stress response? (Consider each of the following: sympathetic stimulation, parasympathetic stimulation, glucocorticoid secretion, and neurogenic vasodilation.)
c. What specific nursing actions promote potassium balance in clients receiving digitalis preparations? (Consider both modification of stress response and dietary management.)
d. How much should clients be told about the risks of drug therapy, such as the danger of cardiac arrest or arterial emboli in response to antiarrhythmic drugs?

2 □ Divide the class into groups of three to eight people for a classroom exercise. Supply each group with data about a client receiving either digitalis or antiarrhythmic drugs. These data are to be used for developing a nursing care plan. After 15 to 20 minutes, bring the groups together to share their plans for nursing care. Client data should include pertinent information about history, medical treatment, and individual response to illness. Situations might include clients with chronic congestive failure, acute heart failure, rheumatic heart disease with atrial fibrillation, and acute digitalis toxicity.

Evaluation Examples (Test Items)

ESSAY QUESTIONS

1. Discuss the relationship between digitalis, calcium and potassium ions, and their effects on the heart.

2. Outline the nursing care required for the client experiencing the signs and symptoms of digitalis toxicity. Include a description of toxic signs and symptoms, specific nursing measures to alter the drug's concentration, and the drug's physiologic action on the heart.

3. What recommendations would you make to a client receiving digitalis therapy for mild, chronic, congestive failure? Assume that a specific diet has not been prescribed, and the client is allowed to eat normally.

MULTIPLE CHOICE ITEMS

1. The digitalis preparation that is eliminated *primarily* through the liver is
1. Digoxin
2. Lanoxin
3. Ouabain
*4. Digitoxin

2. Digoxin has the following effects on heart action:
a. Positive inotropic
b. Positive chronotropic
c. Negative dromotropic
d. Increased automaticity
1. a, b, c
*2. a, c, d
3. a, b, d
4. b, c, d
5. All of the above

3. The normal maintenance dosage for digoxin ranges from
*1. 0.125 mg to 0.25 mg/day
2. 0.25 mg to 0.5 mg/day
3. 1 mg to 1.5 mg/day
4. 2.5 mg to 5 mg/day

4. Foods rich in a nutrient that acts as a physiologic antagonist to digoxin include
a. Apple juice
b. Bananas
c. Whole grain cereals
d. Orange juice
e. Prunes
1. a, b, c
2. a, d, e
*3. b, d
4. c, e
5. All of the above

5. Digitalis toxicity is most likely to develop in clients receiving digitalis in combination with
1. A potassium-sparing diuretic
*2. A potassium-wasting diuretic
3. An oral anticoagulant
4. Potassium supplements

SITUATION-BASED MULTIPLE CHOICE ITEMS

Situation: Mr. HT has been admitted to the hospital with chief complaint of nausea, vomiting, diarrhea, and marked weakness. At home he has been receiving hydrochlorothiazide for hypertension, digoxin for chronic congestive heart failure, and low-dose aspirin for its antiplatelet effect. Data from tests performed the day of admission include the following: electrocardiogram (ECG): narrow QRS complex and prolonged Q–T interval; serum electrolyte concentrations: sodium, 135 mEq/liter; potassium, 3.0 mEq/liter; calcium, 5.0 mEq/liter; serum digoxin concentration, 2.0 mg/ml. A diagnosis of digitalis toxicity has been made.

1. What would you expect the physician to do about the digoxin medication?
1. Continue it at a reduced dosage
*2. Discontinue it for a while
3. Order cathartics to prevent continued absorption of digoxin
4. Order hemodialysis to remove digitalis from the blood

2. Is it likely that the hydrochlorothiazide will be continued?
1. Yes, it is needed to prevent a recurrence of congestive heart failure
2. No, a diuretic would not be necessary until the gastrointestinal upset subsides
*3. No, it is likely that a potassium-sparing diuretic may be ordered in its place
4. No, the hydrochlorothiazide directly sensitizes the myocardium to digoxin

3. How would you interpret a serum digoxin concentration of 2.0 mg/ml?
1. It is indicative of a therapeutic concentration of the digoxin
*2. It is at the level usually designated as beginning toxicity
3. It is above the level usually designated as beginning toxicity
4. It deviates markedly from the expected levels and may be indicative of a laboratory error

4. What is the significance of the serum potassium ion concentration?

a. The client has a low potassium concentration because he has been losing this electrolyte from the gastrointestinal tract
b. The client's kidneys have been retaining some potassium because of stress, causing some increase in this electrolyte's concentration
c. The potassium imbalance is contributing to the toxic reaction to digoxin

1. a only
2. b only
*3. a, c
4. b, c
5. All of the above

5. To assess the degree of digoxin toxicity during treatment, you would

a. Monitor the pulse
b. Monitor the gastrointestinal signs and symptoms
c. Measure the digoxin in blood by a Fingerstix test
d. Monitor the ECG

1. a, b, c
*2. a, b, d
3. a, d, c
4. b, c, d
5. All of the above

6. To monitor changes in the potassium level between blood chemistries, you would

*1. Monitor the client's muscular strength
2. Measure the concentration of potassium in emesis and feces
3. Measure the blood potassium level by a Fingerstix test
4. Monitor the ECG

7. Which of the following would be most indicative of a decrease in the serum digoxin level with persistent hypokalemia?

1. Change to a normal ECG tracing
2. Persistence of nausea and a pulse rate of 104
3. Muscle twitching and spasms
*4. A change from frequent stools and bowel hypermotility to constipation and intestinal atony

8. Following recovery, if HT is discharged on the same medications he took prior to hospitalization, what might he do to prevent a recurrence of digoxin toxicity?

*1. Increase intake of potassium-rich foods
2. Increase intake of calcium-rich foods
3. Increase intake of sodium-rich foods
4. Use a bulk laxative regularly

28 Vascular Drugs

Chapter 28 considers the drugs affecting the peripheral circulation by altering serum lipid levels, influencing vascular tone, or obliterating diseased veins.

Through the study of this chapter, students may develop the following concepts:

1 □ Drugs may be used effectively to alter physiology or treat disease, even though the drugs' specific mechanisms of action are unknown.
2 □ When a new type of drug is introduced, it is usually given first to clients who have failed to respond to the usual therapeutic regimens or who have grave prognoses.
3 □ When a new type of drug is introduced, initial preparations tend to be nonselective and to exhibit many side effects.
4 □ The selectivity of a drug can sometimes be increased by alteration of the chemical molecule (*e.g.*, D-thyronine).
5 □ Substances that act as nutrients in small doses may act as drugs in large doses (*e.g.*, niacin).
6 □ Changes in lifestyle are often more effective than drug therapy in preventing or treating disease.
7 □ Drugs administered transdermally for systemic effect may cause skin irritation (*e.g.*, nitroglycerin ointment).
8 □ Improper storage conditions can inactivate drugs or cause them to become more toxic (*e.g.*, nitroglycerin, sodium nitroprusside).
9 □ Compliance with the drug regimen tends to decrease when a disease is asymptomatic and when the side effects of the drug are discomforting.
10 □ The use of very potent medications requires close monitoring and skilled administration, often in the hospital, to decrease the risk of serious adverse reactions.

Teaching Strategies

1 □ The study of this chapter is best combined with that of Chapters 27, 29, and 38 and integrated in a comprehensive study of cardiovascular disease. Illustrative material can be drawn from the experiences of students and instructors because the diseases treated by these agents, especially abnormalities of blood pressure, are common.
2 □ Topics for class discussion might include the following:

- **a.** The compensatory mechanisms operating in different types of shock (cardiogenic, hypovolemic, and neurogenic) and their implications for the use of vasoconstrictors or vasodilators in the treatment of shock.
- **b.** Recommendations the nurse can make regarding changes in lifestyle that decrease the risk of early cardiovascular disease.
- **c.** Factors influencing motivation to maintain therapeutic regimens (*e.g.*, perceived threat of the disease, discomforting signs and symptoms of the disease, conflicts between the treatment regimen and usual lifestyle, discomforting side effects of the drugs used for treatment, fear of death).

3 □ If a family affected by familial hypercholesterolemia is available in the community, invite a member to attend class and to describe the impact of the condition on the family, and to discuss the measures currently being used to decrease the risk of early cardiovascular disease in young family members.
4 □ Ask a nurse who has undergone treatment for severe or chronic varicose veins to address the class about the signs and symptoms of the disease, its status as an occupational hazard for nurses, treatment regimens, and the long-term effectiveness of treatment.
5 □ Ask a nutritionist to address the class regarding current dietary recommendations to decrease serum lipid levels and to increase the high-density lipoprotein to low-density lipoprotein ratio (HDL:LDL).

Evaluation Examples (Test Items)

ESSAY QUESTIONS

1. Select a subculture characterized by a distinct lifestyle. Describe dietary, drug, and activity customs, and evaluate their impact on the risk of cardiovascular disease.

2. Describe several dietary modifications that are currently believed to reduce the risk of early cardiovascular disease. Explain how each contributes to long-term cardiovascular health.

3. Describe the adverse reactions to antihypertensive drug regimens that may cause reduced compliance with the drug regimen.

4. Identify one drug used in the treatment of varicose veins and describe its pharmacodynamics, methods of administration, toxic and side effects, precautions, and contraindications.

MULTIPLE CHOICE ITEMS

1. The effects that are desired from hypolipidemic therapy include
- a. A decrease in serum triglyceride levels
- b. A decrease in serum HDL levels
- c. A decrease in serum LDL levels
- 1. a, b
- *2. a, c
- 3. b, c
- 4. All of the above
- 5. None of the above

2. Increased cholesterol in the serum is reflected chiefly by increased
- 1. VLDL levels
- *2. LDL levels
- 3. HDL levels
- 4. All of the above
- 5. None of the above; serum cholesterol levels must be measured directly

3. A drug known to lower cholesterol levels in the serum by preventing reabsorption of bile acids in the intestine is
- 1. Clofibrate
- 2. Niacin
- 3. Dextrothyronine
- 4. Ascorbic acid
- *5. Cholestyramine

4. Nitroglycerin sublingual tablets are usually administered
- 1. Twice a day for maintenance effect
- 2. Every 6 hours to maintain blood level
- *3. PRN at 15- to 20-minute intervals
- 4. PRN at 3- to 5-minute intervals

5. An antihypertensive that breaks down readily when exposed to light is
- 1. Nitroglycerin
- *2. Sodium nitroprusside
- 3. Diazoxide
- 4. Trimethadone

6. Effects on the cardiovascular system attributed to vitamin C include
- a. A decrease in capillary fragility
- b. Vasodilation
- c. Acceleration of cholesterol excretion
- 1. a, b
- *2. a, c
- 3. b, c
- 4. All of the above
- 5. None of the above

7. A vasodilator that can produce physical dependence is
- *1. Nitroglycerin
- 2. Hydralazine
- 3. Methyldopa
- 4. Niacin

8. A common side effect of nitroglycerin is
- 1. A transitory rise in blood pressure
- 2. Nausea and vomiting
- 3. A disulfiramlike reaction to use of alcohol
- *4. Headache

9. Nitroglycerin is most often prescribed for the treatment of
- 1. Congestive heart failure
- 2. Hypercholesterolemia
- 3. Hypotension
- *4. Angina pectoris

10 A drug used as a sclerosing agent in the treatment of varicose veins in the legs is
- 1. Lunar caustic
- 2. Sodium tetradecyl
- *3. Sodium morrhuate
- 4. Sodium hydroxide

SITUATION-BASED MULTIPLE CHOICE QUESTIONS

Situation: Mr. AH, age 26 years, has been diagnosed as having hypercholesterolemia. He has been following a low-cholesterol diet for the last 6 months, and his blood cholesterol concentration has declined from 385 mg/dl to 325 mg/dl. The physician has now ordered drug treatment with cholestyramine and niacin in an effort to bring the cholesterol concentration nearer to normal limits.

1. You would anticipate that AH's family history might include
- 1. Long-lived forebears, especially male forebears
- 2. A life expectancy below average, equal in both sexes
- 3. A shortened life expectancy with early onset of cardiovascular disease, especially in women
- *4. A shortened life expectancy with early onset of cardiovascular disease, especially in men

2. Because of his high blood cholesterol concentration, AH is at high risk for
- 1. Atherosclerosis
- 2. Arteriosclerosis
- 3. Hypertension
- *4. All of the above

3. Because cholestyramine contains tartrazine, you should ask Mr. H. specifically about
- 1. Allergy to aspirin
- 2. History of allergic asthma
- 3. History of nasal polyps
- *4. All of the above

4. Instructions for taking cholestyramine should include
- 1. Taking the powder with meals
- *2. Diluting the powder with ample fluids before ingesting
- 3. Taking the cholestyramine and niacin at the same time to decrease the likelihood of missed doses
- 4. All of the above

5. To minimize adverse reactions to cholestyramine, you should teach AH measures to prevent or ameliorate
- 1. Dyspnea
- 2. Hypocalcemia
- *3. Constipation
- 4. Postural hypotension

6. What kind of drug is niacin?
   1. A bile acid-sequestering resin
   2. A hormone
   3. A sympatholytic vasodilator
   *4. A vitamin

7. You would anticipate that the dosage of niacin ordered for AH would be approximately equal to
   1. The minimum daily requirement for nicotinic acid
   2. The amount of nicotinic acid in a therapeutic vitamin preparation
   3. 40 to 50 times the minimum daily requirement for nicotinic acid
   *4. Hundreds of times the minimum daily requirement for nicotinic acid

8. You should advise AH that immediate reactions to niacin in large doses include
   *1. Flushing and itching of the skin
   2. Hypoglycemia
   3. Bradycardia
   4. All of the above

9. AH should know that the use of niacin in pharmacologic doses increases the risk of developing
   1. Gout
   2. Peptic ulcerations
   3. Changes in liver function
   *4. All of the above

Situation: Mr. SW, age 72 years, has been successfully treated for an episode of congestive heart failure. After this illness, his blood pressure was found to be elevated (150-170/90-110). Medication with hydrochlorothiazide reduced the blood pressure somewhat, but the diastolic pressure remained close to 100. Propranolol is now being added to the drug regimen.

1. What kind of drug is propranolol?
   1. A direct vasodilator
   2. A tranquilizer
   3. A nonselective adrenergic blocking agent
   *4. A β-adrenergic blocking agent

2. How often will SW have to take propranolol?
   1. Three or four times daily, because the drug's duration of action is limited
   *2. Once or twice daily, depending on the formulation
   3. Once every day or two, because the drug is formulated as a sustained-release preparation
   4. As required, in relation to the amount of stress SW experiences

3. To minimize adverse reaction to his medications, SW should
   1. Drink ample fluids
   2. Learn to change position slowly
   3. Increase dietary intake of potassium
   *4. All of the above

4. While SW is taking propranolol he is at increased risk for developing
   1. Hypokalemia when under stress
   *2. Hypotension when under stress
   3. Hyperglycemia when under stress
   4. Tachycardia when under stress

5. SW also has a mild diabetes mellitus that is controlled by diet. If he develops a need for insulin he will, because he is taking propranolol, be at increased risk for developing pronounced
   1. Ketoacidosis
   2. Hyperglycemia
   *3. Hypoglycemia
   4. All of the above

6. SW should be cautioned specifically to consult his physician promptly should he develop signs and symptoms of
   1. Postural hypotension
   *2. Congestive heart failure
   3. Sympathetic overstimulation of the heart
   4. Gastrointestinal upset

7. Because he is taking propranolol, SW is at decreased risk for developing
   *1. Angina pectoris
   2. Atherosclerosis
   3. Hypoglycemia
   4. Bronchospasm

8. It would be appropriate to consult SW's physician
   *1. To request parameters for blood pressure desirable for SW
   2. To suggest the prescription of a calcium supplement
   3. To suggest the prescription of emergency prednisone for use if a hypotensive episode occurs during severe stress
   4. To ask if the dietary sodium restriction may be relaxed

9. You would anticipate that desirable blood pressure ranges for SW would most likely be
   1. 100-200/60-70
   2. 120-140/60-80
   *3. 140-150/80-90
   4. 180-200/90-110

Situation: Mr. SC, age 60 years, has been diagnosed as having intermittent mild angina pectoris. His physician has advised sublingual nitroglycerin to control these episodes. You are seeing SC during a home visit for the first time since he was given this prescription.

1. SC tells you he has not had an episode of angina lately and that he has never taken a dose of the nitroglycerin. You might appropriately advise him
   1. Not to take the drug unless he is sure his discomfort is caused by angina
   *2. To take the nitroglycerin as soon as pain likely to be angina occurs
   3. To take the nitroglycerin regularly to maintain vasodilation

2. When you ask to see SC's bottle of medicine, he goes to the bedroom to get it. You should suggest that
   1. SC keep the medicine in his shirt pocket so that it can be taken immediately when angina pain occurs
   *2. SC keep the medicine where it is readily available to him at all times (but not where it will be warmed by body heat)

3. The medication be refrigerated except at times when angina pain is likely to occur

3. SC asks you, "What should I do if the medicine doesn't relieve the pain?" Your best reply would be

1. You should seek emergency medical care promptly
*2. You may take a second or third dose at intervals of 15 to 30 minutes
3. You may take a second or third dose at intervals of 5 to 10 minutes
4. You may take as many doses as necessary as long as they are 30 minutes apart

4. SC should know that, if the pain is persistent, he should

1. Go to bed and rest for at least 4 hours
2. Notify his physician and make an appointment for reevaluation
*3. Call for emergency medical care

5. When should SC renew his nitroglycerin prescription?

1. Only when he has used all of the present prescription
2. Only after seeing his physician for a reevaluation
*3. After 3 months, whether or not all the medicine has been used
4. When the tablets become hardened and fail to dissolve readily

6. SC should be warned that nitroglycerin can cause

a. Weakness and dizziness
b. Severe headache
c. Sexual dysfunction

*1. a, b
2. a, c
3. b, c
4. All of the above

7. To relieve adverse reactions to nitroglycerin, SC may be advised to

1. Lie down and rest quietly for a brief period after taking nitroglycerin
2. Apply cold compresses to the head
3. Take a mild analgesic, such as acetaminophen
*4. All of the above

29
Drugs Affecting Coagulation

Physiology of Coagulation
Pathology
Hemostatics
Systemic Hemostatics
Topical Hemostatics
Nursing Management
Anticoagulants
Heparin
Warfarin
Indanedione Anticoagulants
Drugs That Affect Platelet Aggregation
Nursing Management
Thrombolytic Agents
Nursing Management
Drugs That Enhance Peripheral Circulation
Dimethylsulfoxide and Phytic Acid
Vitamin B_6 Analog
Pentoxifylline
Nursing Management

Chapter 29 describes the delicate balance of blood as a chemical mixture in relationship to coagulation problems and drug administration. Factors and fractional components of blood are reviewed. Inappropriate coagulation is characterized by two types: deficient coagulation and excessive bleeding, and inappropriate coagulation within vessels, which obstructs blood flow. Drug agents used in patients with coagulation problems include substances to restore coagulation, anticoagulants, and agents to dissolve clots.

Through the study of this chapter, the student may develop the following concepts:

1 □ Physiologic responses dependent on a chain of enzymatic reactions can be reduced or impaired by interference with one or more chemical reactions in the chain.
2 □ Interference with a step in enzymatic chain reactions may be a result of an inherited enzyme deficiency or of the action of a drug agent.
3 □ The physiologic effects of an inherited enzyme deficiency may be controlled by administration of blood fractions containing the enzyme factor.
4 □ Drugs made from human blood are limited in supply if they cannot be manufactured synthetically because supply of human blood is limited.
5 □ Blood factors must be carefully handled and stored to maintain their efficacy; they tend to deteriorate when agitated or exposed to extreme temperatures.
6 □ Blood products are a form of tissue transplant and pose some degree of risk because of the transmission of serum hepatitis and AIDS, and because of the incompatibilities of blood type.
7 □ Two drugs with similar physiologic effects, such as heparin and protamine, may be mutually antagonistic if they react to form a stable inactive complex.
8 □ Chemicals that function as essential nutrients in small doses may be toxic in large doses.
9 □ New drugs must be used experimentally on human subjects before they can be approved for general use in medical therapy.
10 □ Clients receiving investigational drugs must be informed of the experimental nature of the treatment before giving informed consent to therapy.
11 □ Drugs with narrow safety margins can sometimes be monitored by means of laboratory blood tests.
12 □ A substance used as a poison may act as an effective medicine if doses are appropriate; close monitoring of client response increases the safety of such use.
13 □ The effect of a drug may be altered by the concurrent administration of other drugs or by the ingestion of certain foods.
14 □ Drugs administered during pregnancy can cross the placenta and affect the fetus.
15 □ Emotional reactions can alter both therapeutic and nontherapeutic responses to medication.
16 □ Drugs of animal origin can induce allergic hypersensitivity in clients receiving them.
17 □ Allergic hypersensitivity to a drug may be temporarily decreased by administering incremental doses of the allergens until therapeutic doses can be tolerated (a technique known as rapid desensitization).
18 □ Clients receiving drugs that alter normal physiology should wear an identification device that specifies the drug in use.

Teaching Strategies

1 □ The mastery of the content of this chapter is greatly enhanced by clinical experience with clients receiving treatment to alter blood coagulation. During the clinical experience, students should monitor laboratory data relating to coagulability, assess clients thoroughly for evidence of abnormal coagulability, and participate in drug administration.
2 □ The study of this chapter may profitability be combined with the study of Chapters 27, 28, and 38 in an integrated unit on cardiovascular disease.
3 □ Develop a chart that lists drugs affecting coagulability, their antidotes (or emergency treatment of toxicity), laboratory tests used to monitor clinical response, and signs and symptoms of toxicity.
4 □ Develop nursing care plans for clients exhibiting hypercoagulability in conditions such as disseminated intravascular coagulation, phlebitis, coronary or

cerebral thrombosis, and hypocoagulability in conditions such as hemophilia or massive transfusions of citrated blood.

Evaluation Examples (Test Items)

ESSAY QUESTIONS

1. List, in order, the steps in the process by which blood clots.

2. Discuss briefly steps in the coagulation process that are impaired in at least three hypocoagulability states.

3. Choose one anticoagulant and one hemostatic drug and for each briefly describe the following: (*a*) the effect the drug has on the coagulation process; (*b*) the method by which therapeutic response to the drug is monitored; (*c*) the antidote or emergency treatment for toxicity; and (*d*) the route by which the drug is commonly administered.

4. Compare and contrast the fibrinolytics streptokinase and tissue plasminogen activator. Consider administration and dosage, duration of effect, side effects, adverse reactions, and cost.

5. Discuss the ethical considerations involved in the administration of experimental drugs to human subjects. Include in your discussion the role of the nurse and ethical dilemmas that may face the nurse participating in the care of clients receiving experimental drugs.

MULTIPLE CHOICE ITEMS

1. The inherited disease caused by a primary deficiency of clotting factor VIII is
 1. Bleeding disease
 2. Hageman disease
 3. Christmas disease
 *4. Hemophilia

2. The emergency treatment for excessive bleeding caused by massive transfusions of citrated blood is
 1. Vitamin K, given by injection
 2. Intravenous administration of protamine sulfate
 3. Intravenous administration of clotting factor VIII
 *4. Intravenous administration of calcium

3. Treatment for excessive bleeding caused by hemophilia involves
 1. Protamine sulfate, administered orally
 *2. Intravenous administration of clotting factor VIII
 3. Intravenous administration of calcium
 4. Blood transfusion; no other treatment is effective

4. To preserve its efficacy, antihemophilic factor should be
 1. Stored in a warm dry place
 2. Stored in a cool dry room
 *3. Stored in a refrigerator
 4. Frozen quickly and stored at 0°F

5. Blood and blood products can cause complications because of
 a. Incompatibility of blood types
 b. Transmission of serum hepatitis virus
 1. a only
 2. b only
 *3. a, b
 4. Neither a nor b

6. Dietary sources of large amounts of vitamin K include
 a. Citrus fruits
 b. Green leafy vegetables
 c. Liver
 1. a, b
 2. a, c
 *3. b, c
 4. All of the above

7. Because it can cause toxic symptoms, vitamin K must be administered with caution to
 *1. Infants
 2. Pregnant women
 3. Clients subject to hemophilia
 4. Elderly clients

8. Vitamin K is the antidote for
 1. Heparin
 2. Hyperprothrombinemia
 3. Fibrinogen
 *4. Warfarin

9. The antidote for heparin is
 1. Vitamin A
 2. Vitamin D
 3. Calcium
 *4. Protamine sulfate

10. Heparin is usually administered
 a. Orally
 b. Subcutaneously
 c. Intramuscularly
 d. Intravenously
 1. a, b
 2. c, d
 3. a, c
 *4. b, d
 5. All of the above

11. Epinephrine slows bleeding primarily by
 1. Stimulating the production of clotting factors
 2. Stimulating the release of clotting factors
 3. Replacing one or more clotting factors
 *4. Inducing vasoconstriction

12. Thrombin is administered
 *1. Topically
 2. Orally
 3. Subcutaneously
 4. Intravenously

13. Thrombin acts to stop bleeding by
 1. Stimulating the production of clotting factors
 2. Stimulating the release of clotting factors

*3. Replacing one or more clotting factors
4. Inducing vasoconstriction

14. When packs that have been impregnated with hemostatics are to be removed from body cavities such as the nose or vagina, they must first be
1. Soaked with thrombin solution to inhibit bleeding
*2. Soaked with saline solution to prevent tissue damage
3. Soaked with warfarin solution to dissolve clots that cause them to adhere to the tissues
4. Soaked with a disinfectant to prevent infection

15. Select the answer that best describes statements a and b:
a. Bleeding tendencies are more dangerous than hypercoagulable states
b. When anticoagulants are administered, great care must be taken to prevent serum concentrations from reaching toxic levels; it is better to undertreat than to overtreat
1. a and b are both true, and a helps to explain b
2. a and b are both true, but a does not help to explain b
3. a is true but b is false
4. a is false but b is true
*5. Both a and b are false

16. An anticoagulant drug used as a rodenticide is
1. Thrombin
2. Heparin
3. Ascorbic acid
*4 Warfarin

17. A drug that interacts with warfarin by inhibiting its absorption in the gastrointestinal tract is
1. Phenobarbital
*2. Griseofulvin
3. Vitamin K
4. Phenylbutazone

18. The laboratory test used to evaluate response to warfarin therapy is
*1. Prothrombin time
2. Partial thromboplastin time
3. Bleeding time
4. Vitamin K titer

SITUATION-BASED MULTPLE CHOICE ITEMS

Situation: Ms. TR, age 43 years, is being admitted to your hospital nursing unit from the emergency room with a diagnosis of acute thrombophlebitis of the right leg. She is to receive both heparin and coumarin anticoagulants.

1. To prepare for the administration of heparin, you would
1. Locate the stock bottle of oral heparin tablets
2. Locate the stock bottle of injectable heparin solution and assemble equipment for an intramuscular injection
*3. Assemble tubing and a control device for an intravenous infusion

2. Before administering the first doses of anticoagulants, you should ask TR if she has
a. Received heparin or coumarin in the past
b. An allergy to fish
c. An allergy to heparin or coumarin
1. a, b
2. a, c
3. b, c
*4. All of the above

3. You would inform TR that she can expect to
a. Be on complete bed rest
b. Have blood drawn each morning for laboratory tests
c. Develop black and blue areas over many areas of the body
*1. a, b
2. a, c
3. b, c
4. All of the above

4. The second day of TR's hospitalization, the physician changed the heparin dosage and ordered the medication to be given subcutaneously every 3 hours. You would administer these injections into the
1. Fat pad over the ventrogluteal area, massaging well after injection
2. Fat pad over the ventrogluteal area, aspirating carefully before depressing the plunger of the syringe
3. Subcutaneous tissue over the deltoid muscle, observing standard precautions for injections
*4. Fat pads of the abdomen without aspirating or massaging

5. To prevent an adverse reaction to the anticoagulants, you should
*1. Warn TR to avoid trauma such as razor cuts
2. Warn TR to avoid any physical exertion
3. Order a diet rich in vitamin K
4. Do all of the above

6. To detect early anticoagulant toxicity, you should monitor TR's
1. Vital signs frequently
2. Stools for frank blood
*3. Urine for discoloration
4. Level of consciousness

7. If TR begins to hemorrhage, which of the following is likely to be used to treat the bleeding?
1. Antihemophilia factor
*2. Whole blood or blood plasma
3. Factor IX complex
4. Vitamin K_1

8. What is the specific antidote for heparin?
1. Vitamine K_1
2. Thrombin
3. Factor IX complex
*4. Protamine sulfate

9. You would anticipate that, during about the middle of the first week of treatment,
1. The coumarin will be discontinued

*2. The heparin will be discontinued
3. Both anticoagulants will be discontinued
4. Small doses of both protamine sulfate and vitamin K_1 will be given to prevent abnormal bleeding

10. What laboratory test is used to monitor coumarin anticoagulation?
1. Erythrocyte sedimentation rate (ESR)
2. Partial thromboplastin time (PTT)
*3. Prothrombin time (PT)
4. Lee White clotting time

Situation: Ms. EB has been admitted to the hospital with a diagnosis of menorrhagia of 10 weeks' duration. She has a hemoglobin concentration of 7 g/dl and appears pale and weak. Her physician has unsuccessfully tried hormone injections in the office to terminate the bleeding.

1. Whole blood transfusions are being ordered for EB to
a. Slow or stop the bleeding
b. Raise the hemoglobin concentration
c. Replenish clotting factors that may be deficient
1. a, b
2. a, c
3. b, c
*4. All of the above

2. Of the following drugs, which is most likely to be ordered as an adjunct to treatment?
1. Protamine sulfate
2. Vitamin K_1
*3. Ferrous gluconate
4. Vitamin A

3. TB's bleeding decreases somewhat in severity but continues. A diagnostic work-up indicates that she is probably suffering from a form of Christmas disease. You would anticipate that the physician might next order
1. One or more units of blood plasma
2. Antihemophilia factor
*3. Factor IX complex
4. All of the above

4. You may reassure TB that the new treatment will probably
1. Return clotting to normal and stop the vaginal flow
*2. Markedly decrease the bleeding and improve clotting
3. Arrest the bleeding disorder and produce a long-term remission
4. Restore hemoglobin levels to normal

UNIT SEVEN: DRUGS AFFECTING THE GASTROINTESTINAL SYSTEM

30 Agents Affecting the Upper Gastrointestinal Tract

Agents Used for the Mouth
- *Physiology of the Upper GI Tract*
- *Pathology of the Upper GI Tract*
- *Dentifrices*
- *Nursing Management for Dentifrices*
- *Mouthwashes and Gargles*
- *Nursing Management for Mouthwashes*

Digestants
- *Physiology*
- *Pathology*
- *Gastric Acidifiers*
- *Digestive Enzymes*
- *Bile and Bile Acids*
- *Nursing Management*

Drug Therapy for Disorders Associated with Hyperacidity
- *Physiology*
- *Pathology*
- *Drugs Used to Suppress Acid Production*
- *Antacids*
- *Sucralfate*
- *Nursing Management*

Antiemetics
- *Pathophysiology*
- *Drugs Used to Control Vomiting*
- *Nursing Management*

Emetics
- *Apomorphine*
- *Ipecac*
- *Nursing Management*

Chapter 30 presents material on medicinal and hygienic substances used for their effects on the upper gastrointestinal tract. These include drugs employed to control hyperacidity, nausea, and vomiting. Hygienic aids include such self-care products as toothpastes and mouthwashes. Because many medicinal substances are available as over-the-counter remedies, there is considerable material related to self-care practices and the need to advise and inform clients regarding self-medication.

Most of the substances discussed in this chapter are palliative rather than curative in nature. The value of control of symptoms to supplement supportive measures while the body heals itself could be emphasized during study of this portion of the textbook.

Among the drugs discussed are the histamine-2 receptor antagonists, which are relatively new treatment agents. These have generated so much enthusiasm that cimetidine currently is one of the most frequently prescribed medications, despite the fact that little is known about its long-term adverse effects.

Through study of the chapter, students may develop the following concepts:

1 □ Self-medication is appropriate for many short-term, self-limiting conditions, provided symptoms are not severe; when using over-the-counter preparations for control of minor illnesses, clients should use the least amount that is effective and the least toxic substance available.

2 □ If symptoms of self-medicated illness are severe or prolonged, medical care should be sought.

3 □ The cost of medicines influences compliance and the degree of stress the illness imposes on the client; nurses should be aware of costs and assist clients to minimize them.

4 □ Adverse reactions to new drugs are not fully identified until they have been widely used for a number of years (10 to 20, or more); nurses should carefully assess responses to these drugs to help clarify the nature of toxic and side effects.

5 □ Palliative drugs perform important functions and complement general supportive measures designed to promote spontaneous recovery from conditions for which there is no definitive cure.

6 □ Drugs ordered to be given as needed (PRN) may be administered prior to development of symptoms, if necessary to the management of the condition.

7 □ Supposedly inactive components of drugs (such as mineral cations in antacids) can cause side effects in some clients.

Teaching Strategies

1 □ Classroom activities might include discussion of the following topics:

a. Impact of medication cost on client compliance.

b. The influence that third-party payment has on choice of treatment regimens.

c. General measures for the treatment of poisoning: use of emetics, gastric lavage, general supportive measures.

d. The effects of supposedly inert components of medicinal agents (*e.g.*, the metallic cations in antacids).

e. Popularity of specific drugs and the influence of the prescriber's preference on prescription practices (especially in relation to a new drug whose effectiveness is apparent before its toxic and side effects are identified).

f. Delayed effects of drugs (*e.g.*, teratogenicity in relation to thalidomine).

2 □ Individual learning activities suggested in the textbook could be used as a basis for additional classroom activities:

a. A debate on the question, "Should fluoride salts be added to supplies of drinking water in areas in which natural fluoride levels are low?"

b. Development of criteria for evaluating advertisements for over-the-counter drugs and hygienic aids.

c. Development of guidelines for use of fluorine supplements.

d. A discussion of traditional remedies (folk medicine) and nursing approaches in working with clients who rely on such practices.

e. Discussion of specific techniques for assessing gastrointestinal symptoms.

Evaluation Examples (Test Items)

MULTIPLE CHOICE ITEMS

1. The use of bile acids is contraindicated for clients with

1. An intolerance to dietary fats
2. A tendency toward constipation
3. A tendency toward diarrhea

*4. Complete biliary obstruction

2. Magnesium antacids tend to cause

1. Constipation

*2. Diarrhea

3. Nephrotoxicity
4. Hypertension

SITUATION-BASED MULTIPLE CHOICE ITEMS

Situation: As a public health nurse, you are caring for a family whose husband and father, Mr. NU (a 31-year-old truck driver), has been diagnosed as having a peptic ulcer in the bulb of the duodenum. His physician has ordered a bland diet, cimetidine (Tagamet) 300 mg qid, and aluminum hydroxide gel (Amphojel) for epigastric pain.

1. NU's wife is shocked at the cost of cimetidine and asks you if it is really necessary to use this new drug. Appropriate replies would be that

a. Over-the-counter antacids and ranitidine can also be used to treat peptic ulcer, and the family could consult the physician about alternative regimens

b. Cimetidine causes fewer and less serious adverse reactions than do alternative medications

c. Over-the-counter antacids are usually not paid for by insurance plans that cover prescription medication

d. The use of alternative medication is likely to be at least as expensive as cimetidine over the course of treatment

1. a, b, c
2. a, b, d

*3. a, c, d

4. b, c, d
5. All of the above

2. After the first week of treatment, NU is still experiencing epigastric distress before meals. He admits that he is not taking Amphojel for this discomfort while working because, the first day that he took the medication to work, the bottle was accidentally broken. He asks you why he cannot use Amphojel tablets when away from home. You would advise him that

1. His ulcer is unlikely to heal unless he uses a liquid medication consistently

*2. The tablets are helpful but are not as effective as the liquid preparation

3. The tablets may be substituted for the liquid preparation, because they are as effective as the liquid medication
4. If he uses tablets, he should switch to Maalox, because these tablets are less constipating than Amphojel

3. If NU decides to use oral tablets, how would you advise him to take them

1. Swallow them whole with no more than 4 ounces of liquid
2. Swallow them whole with a full glass of liquid
3. Chew them thoroughly and follow with a full glass of liquid

*4. Chew them thoroughly or suck on them so that they disintegrate before swallowing

4. After a month of treatment, NU feels better, but his wife confides that he is not taking his medicine as often as the doctor had prescribed because he has heard that cimetidine can make him "less manly." You should tell them that

1. Cimetidine has no effect on sexuality

*2. Cimetidine sometimes affects male sexuality and that, if it does, NU should ask the physician for a reevaluation of the drug regimen

3. NU is getting along satisfactorily on less medication, and need not change the way he is taking his medicine
4. NU should increase his use of antacids to compensate for using less cimetidine

5. Two months later, the physician advises NU to decrease his dosage of cimetidine gradually, dropping one dose at a time. Which dose should be continued the longest?

1. The dose taken after breakfast
2. The dose taken after lunch
3. The dose taken after dinner
* 4. The bedtime dose

6. NU has developed an increasing problem with constipation. You would advise him to
   a. Ask the physician if he can use a less constipating antacid
   b. Drink plenty of fluids
   c. Add bran to his diet
   d. Set aside a regular time each day for defecation
   1. a, b, c
   *2. a, b, d
   3. a, c, d
   4. b, c, d
   5. All of the above

31
Agents Affecting the Lower Gastrointestinal Tract

Antiflatulents
  Pathophysiology
  Carminatives
  Simethicone
  Nursing Management
Drugs Affecting Fecal Elimination
  Physiology
  Pathophysiology
  Laxatives
Antidiarrheals
  Pathophysiology
  Agents Used in the Treatment of Diarrhea
  Nursing Management

Chapter 31 presents material on prescription and nonprescription drugs employed for their effects on the lower gastrointestinal tract. These include antiflatulents, laxatives, and antidiarrheals. There is considerable material related to self-care practices and the need to advise and inform clients regarding self-medication.

Most of the drugs discussed in this chapter are palliative rather than curative in nature. The value of symptom control and supportive measures while the body heals itself could be emphasized during study of this portion of the text.

Through the study of this chapter, students may develop the following concepts:

1 □ Self-medication is appropriate for many short-term, self-limiting conditions, provided symptoms are not severe; when using over-the-counter preparations for control of minor illnesses, clients should use the least amount that is effective and the least toxic substance available.
2 □ If symptoms of self-medicated illness are severe or prolonged, medical care should be sought.
3 □ Palliative drugs perform important functions and complement general supportive measures designed to promote spontaneous recovery from conditions for which there is no definitive cure.
4 □ Tendencies toward constipation or diarrhea are best controlled by hygienic measures—diet, exercise, rest, and habit formation; reliance on drugs alters natural rhythms, tends to perpetuate problems, and can lead to drug dependence.
5 □ Supposedly inactive components of drugs (such as mineral cations in antacids) can cause side effects in some clients.

Teaching Strategies

1 □ Classroom activities might include discussion of the following topics:
  a. Hygienic measures likely to promote fecal elimination in clients with a tendency toward constipation.
  b. Hygienic measures likely to reduce the frequency of stools and fecal loss of fluids in clients with a tendency toward diarrhea.
  c. Criteria for referral to a physician for definitive diagnosis of conditions associated with constipation. (Or for diagnosis of conditions associated with diarrhea.)
  d. Significance of alternating constipation and diarrhea as a symptom of malignancy, diverticulosis or diverticulitis, and chronic use of laxatives.
2 □ Individual learning activities suggested in the textbook could be used as a basis for additional classroom activities:
  a. Discussion of traditional remedies (folk medicine) and nursing approaches in working with clients who rely on such practices.
  b. Discussion of specific techniques for assessing gastrointestinal symptoms.
  c. Developing guidelines for making choices among different kinds of laxative products when the use of laxatives is appropriate.
  d. Development of a teaching program designed to aid a client with a tendency toward constipation to establish optimal bowel habits.

Evaluation Examples (Test Items)

MULTIPLE CHOICE ITEMS

1. A home remedy used as a carminative is essence of
  1. Cloves
  2. Cinnamon
  3. Anise
  *4. Peppermint

2. A folk remedy for diarrhea is
  1. Coffee
  2. Grape wine
  *3. Elderberry wine
  4. Whiskey

SITUATION-BASED MULTIPLE CHOICE ITEMS

Situation: Your neighbor calls one morning to ask you what she should take for a "stomach bug." She is experiencing stomach cramps, and had three loose stools during the night. You are aware that there have recently been several cases of a short-term ("24-hour") gastrointestinal upset among the neighbors.

1. Before recommending an over-the-counter antidiarrheal medication, you should rule out

1. Watery stools
2. Localized pain in the right lower quadrant
3. Dehydration
*4. Fever

2. An over-the-counter medication likely to be effective in reducing your neighbor's discomfort is

1. Aluminum hydroxode (Amphojel)
*2. Kaopectate (kaolin with pectin)
3. Magnesium and aluminum hydroxide (Maalox)
4. Milk of magnesia

3. You would caution your neighbor to consult a physician if her symptoms persist for more than

*1. 1 day
2. 3 days
3. 1 week
4. 2 weeks

4. Other symptoms that signal the need to consult a physician would be

1. An abrupt cessation of stools and abdominal pain
*2. A feeling of pronounced faintness and weakness
3. Weight gain and tissue edema
4. Anorexia accompanied by thirst

5. Your neighbor has a 9-month-old baby. She should know that, if the baby develops diarrhea, she should

1. Give the child a reduced dose of the over-the-counter medicine
2. Withhold food and fluids until the diarrhea abates
3. Give the baby weak coffee to drink
*4. Take the child to a physician without delay

UNIT EIGHT: DRUGS AFFECTING THE ENDOCRINE SYSTEM

32 Steroid Hormones and Their Antagonists

Nature of Hormones
Biological Measurement Techniques
Dosage Regimens
Steroid Hormones
The Steroid Nucleus
Corticosteroids
Glucocorticoids
Mineralocorticoids
Male Sex Hormones
Androgens
Male Hormone Antagonists
Female Sex Hormones
Estrogens
Antiestrogens
Progestogens

Chapter 32 discusses adrenal corticosteroids (glucocorticosteroids and mineralocorticosteroids) and sex hormones and their antagonists.

Through the study of this chapter, the students may develop the following concepts:

1 □ Chemical interactions in the body are extremely complex; they involve multiple interrelationships among autogenous biochemicals, exogenous drugs, foods, and other environmental substances.
2 □ Hormone imbalances tend to be multiple; because of the interrelatedness of the endocrine glands, alteration of levels of one hormone often cause secondary changes in levels of other hormones.
3 □ Hormones are extremely potent chemicals; dosages of pure hormones are often measured in microgram doses.
4 □ Bioassay techniques allow accurate administration of doses measured in units, even when the drugs are not refined or when their active ingredients are unknown.
5 □ The need for hormones varies among people and in the same person over time; it is influenced by environmental factors such as diet and stress, and by internal factors, including biologic rhythms, reproductive status, and illness.
6 □ Hormones affect many fundamental processes in the body: metabolism, immunity, fluid and electrolyte balance, growth and development, healing, and reproduction.
7 □ Changing the molecular structure of a hormone drug can increase its selectivity but side effects cannot be eliminated completely.
8 □ Successful therapy with hormones and hormone antagonists requires careful and continuous monitoring of hormone balance and response to the drugs.
9 □ Active participation by clients in their therapeutic regimens is critical for the management of chronic conditions involving hormone therapy.
10 □ Use of hormones and hormone antagonists tends to require therapy over a long period of time—often for life.
11 □ Physical dependence on hormones may occur when hormone drugs trigger negative feedback systems controlling endocrine function and cause atrophy of secreting glands; when this occurs, clients must be withdrawn gradually (weaned) from drug regimens.
12 □ Timing of drug doses is critical to effective therapy (*e.g.*, alternate-day regimen for long-term prednisone therapy, administration of replacement hormones to mimic diurnal rhythms, synchronization of hormone therapy with the menstrual cycle).
13 □ Hormone imbalances tend to be insidious in onset. Toxicity to hormone and hormone antagonists also develops insidiously. Assessment skills of the nurse are critical to early detection of problems.
14 □ Pronounced hormone imbalances produce medical crises that are life-threatening.

Teaching Strategies

Content on hormone drugs is included in Chapters 33, 34, 36 and in the portion of Chapter 22 dealing with the sympathetic nervous system. Material on the glucocorticosteroids and epinephrine may be assigned in relation to units of study dealing with adaptation to stress. Integration of this content with material dealing with psychological, spiritual, and cultural reactions to stress will assist students to view clients and their problems more holistically.

1 □ To understand drug therapy affecting hormone balance, students need a thorough knowledge of the anatomy and physiology of the endocrine system. Students should be directed to review this content as necessary prior to and during the study of this chapter. The interrelationships between endocrine structures and hormones, and the mechanisms controlling function of this system, are of particular importance.
2 □ Because of the complexity of the endocrine system, it is difficult to organize the progression of learning from the simple to the complex. However, early class discussions could center on the mineralocorticoids, because their levels are not altered markedly by pituitary tropic hormones.

3 □ If time for considering hormone drugs is limited, it is suggested that study focus on the glucocorticoids as examples illustrating the following properties of hormones: (*a*) the effects of these hormones on physiologic function is pervasive—imbalances affect physical appearance, mental and emotional function, fluid and electrolyte balance, energy metabolism, resistance to disease, and circulation; (*b*) environmental factors markedly influence individual needs for this hormone—dosage requirements are variable from client to client and in the same person from time to time; (*c*) natural production of the hormone follows a distinctive diurnal rhythm, which should be reproduced during replacement therapy; (*d*) glucocorticoids are frequently prescribed for a pharmacologic effect; (*e*) glucocorticoid secretion is stimulated by a pituitary tropic hormone, ACTH—maintenance of hormone balance involves a negative feedback mechanism; (*f*) prolonged administration of glucocorticoids inhibits ACTH production, causing atrophy of the adrenals and physiologic dependence on the hormone drug.

A detailed study of the glucocorticoids assists students to understand many physiologic responses to stress, and can enrich the stress adaptation content in the nursing curriculum.

Evaluation Examples (Test Items)

ESSAY QUESTIONS

1. Briefly identify and discuss factors influencing glucose balance in clients receiving insulin therapy.

2. Identify and describe briefly the physiologic effects of glucocorticoid excess.

MULTIPLE CHOICE ITEMS

1. Most hormone drugs that are administered by mouth are
 1. Salts
 2. Proteins
 *3 Steroids
 4. Iodinated amines

2. When glucocorticoids are administered as replacement therapy, what adjustments in dosage are required to compensate for environmental factors affecting hormone need?
 1. Dosage is increased in accord with increased dietary intake
 2. Five to fifteen extra units are administered, depending on results of urine glucose tests
 3. Dosage is decreased by a third to a half when environmental stress stimulates endogenous stress hormone secretion
 *4. Dosage is increased twofold to threefold according to the level of environmental stress

3. The physiologic effects of prednisone include
 a. Hypoglycemia
 b. A tendency to develop peptic ulcers
 c. A tendency to develop diabetes mellitus
 d. Delayed coagulation
 e. Inhibition of the growth of pathogenic microorganisms
 f. Reduction in the inflammatory response
 1. a, b
 *2. b, c, f
 3. c, d, e
 4. a, d, e
 5. f only

4. By what routes is oxycorticosterone administered?
 a. Oral
 b. Intramuscular
 c. Pellet implantation
 1. a, b
 *2. b, c
 3. a, c
 4. All of the above
 5. None of the above

5. Anabolic androgens are approved for medicinal use to
 *1. Stimulate tissue rebuilding in debilitating diseases
 2. Increase muscle mass in professional athletes
 3. Replace male sex hormones in deficient postpubertal men
 4. Stimulate sexual maturation in cases of male hormone deficiency

6. Estrogen replacement hormone therapy of postmenopausal women is avoided whenever possible because maintenance of high estrogen levels for prolonged periods after menopause increases the risk of
 1. Infertility
 2. Osteoporosis
 3. Cardiovascular disease
 *4. Uterine malignancies

7. Side effects of estrogen administration to men include
 a. Genital atrophy
 b. Impotency
 c. Gynecomastia
 1. a, b
 2. b, c
 3. a, c
 *4. All of the above
 5. None of the above

8. The preferred treatment of dyspareunia caused by vaginal atrophy in postmenopausal women is
 1. Avoidance of intercourse
 *2. Topical lubricants applied vaginally prior to intercourse
 3. Topical estrogen creams applied vaginally following intercourse
 4. Systemic estrogens to supply complete hormone replacement

9. Fluctuation in therapeutic response to mineralocorticoids may be minimized by manipulation of the intake of
 a. Carbohydrates
 b. Fluids
 c. Potassium
 d. Sodium

1. a, b
*2. c, d
3. a, c, d
4. b only
5. All of the above

SITUATION-BASED MULTIPLE CHOICE ITEMS

Situation: As a public health nurse, you are caring for Mr. PB, a 17-year-old receiving prednisone 10 mg tid for the treatment of retinitis caused by focusing on an eclipse of the sun. It is expected that drug therapy will continue for at least a year to minimize lasting effects on vision.

1. The desired therapeutic action of the drug in this situation is most likely to be
1. Reduction of edema in the injured area by decreasing sodium retention
2. Prevention of stress-induced hypovolemic shock
*3. Suppression of inflammation and scarring
4. Prevention of abnormal clotting in the eye

2. Among the side effects likely to develop as treatment continues are
a. Loss of weight and thinning of the torso
b. Rounding of the face and thinning of the extremities
c. Hypotension and a tendency toward shock
d. A lowered serum potassium level and decreased resistance to infection
1. a, b, c
2. a, c
*3. b, d
4. d only
5. All of the above

3. You should teach PB
a. To limit his intake of calcium-rich foods and to increase his use of salt
b. To eat a diet moderate in calories and rich in potassium
c. To avoid exposure to infection
d. Techniques to promote sleep at night
1. a, b, c
2. a, b, d
3. a, c, d
*4. b, c, d
5. All of the above

4. The prednisone prescription may be changed at a later date, with instructions that the drug be taken
1. Regularly, around the clock
2. Every day, on arising
3. Every day, on retiring
*4. Every other day, on arising

5. Before beginning the course of prednisone treatment, PB should be informed that he may
a. Notice mood changes while taking the drug
b. Experience daytime drowsiness on the day he takes the drug
c. Notice changes in his appearance after taking the drug for a time
d. Stop growing while taking the drug
1. a, b, c
2. a, b, d
*3. a, c, d
4. b, c, d
5. All of the above

33

Protein Hormones: Insulin and Other Drugs Affecting Blood Glucose

Insulin
Oral Hypoglycemics
Hyperglycemics

Chapter 33 discusses drugs that influence blood glucose levels. A knowledge of these drugs is essential to every nurse because of the high incidence of diabetes mellitus, a chronic disease that contributes greatly to morbidity and mortality in developed countries.

Through the study of this chapter, students may develop the following concepts:

1 □ Chemical interactions in the body are extremely complex; they involve multiple interrelationships among autogenous biochemicals, exogenous drugs, foods, and other environmental substances.

2 □ Hormone imbalances tend to be multiple; because of the interrelatedness of the endorcrine glands, alteration of levels of one hormone often cause secondary changes in levels of other hormones.

3 □ Hormones are extremely potent chemicals: dosages of pure hormones are often measured in microgram doses.

4 □ Bioassay techniques allow accurate administration of doses measured in units, even when the drugs are not refined or when their active ingredients are unknown.

5 □ The need for hormones varies among people and in the same person over time; it is influenced by environmental factors such as diet, stress, and internal factors, including biologic rhythms, reproductive status, and illness.

6 □ Hormones affect many fundamental processes in the body: metabolism, fluid and electrolyte balance, and growth and development.

7 □ Successful therapy with hormones and hormone antagonists requires careful and continuous monitoring of hormone balance and response to the drugs.

8 □ Active participation by clients in their therapeutic regimens is critical for the management of chronic conditions involving hormone therapy.

9 □ Use of hormones and hormone antagonists tends to require therapy over a long period of time—often for life.

10 □ Timing of drug doses is critical to effective therapy (*e.g.*, tailoring dosage of hypoglycemics to the client's rest/activity and eating routines).

11 □ Hormone imbalances tend to be insidious in onset. Toxicity to hormone and hormone antagonists also develops insidiously. Assessment skills of the nurse are critical to early detection of problems.

12 □ Pronounced hormone imbalances produce medical crises that are life-threatening.

13 □ Drugs of animal origin tend to be antigenic to humans.

14 □ Genetic engineering techniques may provide more plentiful supplies of human-specific hormones with reduced antigenic potential.

15 □ Protein hormones must be carefully stored and handled to prevent deterioration.

16 □ Hormone drugs are often marketed as depot preparations that are absorbed slowly.

Teaching Strategies

If the curriculum includes a comprehensive study of endocrine diseases and drugs acting as hormones, Chapter 33 may be assigned to students along with Chapters 32, 34, 36, and the portion of Chapter 22 dealing with the sympathomimetic drugs epinephrine and norepinephrine.

1 □ To understand drug therapy affecting hormone balance, students need a thorough knowledge of the anatomy and physiology of the endocrine system. Students should be directed to review this content as necessary prior to and during the study of this chapter. The interrelationships between endocrine structures and hormones, and the mechanisms controlling function of this system, are of particular importance.

2 □ Because of the complexity of the endocrine system, it is difficult to organize the progression of learning from the simple to the complex. Early class discussions could center on insulin and glucagon, however, as examples of hormones whose levels are more responsive to blood chemistry (glucose level) than to other hormones. They appear not to be influenced by pituitary tropic hormones.

3 □ The study of insulin involves consideration of concepts common to many other hormone preparations, including the following: (*a*) its effects are influenced by environmental factors such as food intake and stress level; (*b*) it is measured in biologic units rather than in weight of pure drug; (*c*) insulin is often modified to delay absorption and physiologic effects; (*d*) insulin is a protein substance that must be stored and handled carefully; (*e*) insulin is administered to most clients for the purpose of hormone replacement; (*f*) insulin therapy is usually continued over long periods of time, often for life; (*g*) active client involvement in the therapeutic regimen is critical for successful long-term insulin therapy; (*h*) pharmaceutic insulin is derived from animal tissues or bacterial cultures and functions as an antigen that stimulates allergic sensitivity in some clients.

Evaluation Examples (Test Items)

ESSAY QUESTION

1. In relation to the mutually antagonistic hormones insulin and glucagon, discuss in detail the effects each has on physiology, the mechanisms controlling their secretion, and the signs and symptoms of imbalance. Identify the organ(s) involved in production of these hormones.

MULTIPLE CHOICE ITEMS

1. Insulin preparations that can be added to glucose solutions for intravenous administration are distinguishable from other insulin preparations by

1. Their origin as products of recombinant DNA techniques
2. Their origin as biological products of animal slaughter or bacterial cultures
3. Their duration of action, which is prolonged by addition of a metallic ion
*4. Their solubility as shown by the clarity of the solution

2. Following successful treatment of hypoglycemia with glucagon, most clients should be given

1. Sugar, candy or jelly to eat
*2. A meat sandwich or crackers and cheese to eat
3. A fatty food such as artificially sweetened ice cream
4. Low-calorie fluids such as dietetic Kool-Aid

3. The wife of an insulin-dependent diabetic asks you, "What should I do if my husband appears to be ill but I cannot tell whether he has high or low blood glucose?" Your best reply is

1. Delay treatment until the signs and symptoms clearly indicate the problem
2. Treat both possible problems by administering food and insulin
3. Administer insulin to prevent dangerous hyperglycemia
*4. Administer food to prevent dangerous hypoglycemia

SITUATION-BASED MULTIPLE CHOICE ITEMS

Situation: Mrs. DM has responded well to treatment for diabetic ketoacidosis during her 6-day hospital stay. She has recovered from the infection that precipitated the episode, and is to be discharged as soon as she has been stabilized on a new regimen of insulin and diet. For the past 2 days she has been on a 1500-calorie ADA diet and receiving 20 units NPH (Isophane) insulin before breakfast daily, with regular insulin coverage for ac or hs glycosuria.

1. When NPH insulin is administered once daily, before breakfast, hypoglycemic reactions are most likely to occur

a. 2 hours after the drug is injected
b. At midday (before lunch)
c. Before the third meal of the day (supper)
d. Before bedtime
e. During sleep (in the early morning hours)
1. a, b
*2. c, d
3. a, e
4. b, c, d
5. e only

2. Factors that reduce body need for insulin include

a. Exercise
b. Reduction in stress levels
c. Interrupted therapy
1. a only
*2. a, b
3. b, c
4. c only
5. None of the above—the need for insulin is affected only by the level of pancreatic islet function and calorie intake

3. While you are making rounds at the beginning of the evening shift (4 PM), DM complains of a headache and slight nausea. When taking her pulse, you note that her hand trembles slightly and feels cool and moist. It is most likely that DM is experiencing

1. A relapse into ketoacidosis
*2. An insulin reaction
3. Respiratory alkalosis from hyperventilation
4. None of the above—there are insufficient data given to indicate the problem

4. In preparation for discharge, it would be appropriate to teach DM that

a. Changes in stress levels can alter glucose balance and response to insulin
b. Exercise decreases the risk of insulin reaction
c. The bedtime snack provided in her diet will help prevent insulin reactions in the early night hours
1. a, b
*2. a, c
3. b, c
4. All of the above

5. The day DM is to be discharged, she is notified that her husband is in the emergency room after experiencing chest pain at work. Her reaction to this sudden stressor is likely to

a. Increase the risk of insulin reaction
b. Increase the risk of hyperglycemia
c. Increase the risk of hyperventilation
1. a, b
2. a only
*3. b, c
4. c only
5. All of the above

34 Thyroid, Parathyroid, Pituitary, and Hypothalamic Hormones

Proteinaceous Hormones
- *Thyroid Hormones*
- *Antithyroid Drugs*
- *Thioamides*
- *Iodine*
- *Radioiodine*
- *Calcitonin*
- *Parathyroid Hormone*

Adenohypophyseal Hormones and Related Substances
- *Adrenocorticotropic Hormone*
- *Growth Hormone*
- *Thyrotropin*

Hypothalamic Hormones
- *Antidiuretic Hormone*
- *Oxytocin*

Chapter 34 discusses the proteinaceous hormones of the thyroid, parathyroid, pituitary, and hypothalamus, and antithyroid drugs. The workbook has exercises on this material; in addition, there are in the workbook a group of exercises relating to hormones in general, to be worked after the student has completed Chapters 32, 33, and 34.

Through the study of this chapter, students may develop the following concepts:

1 ☐ Chemical interactions in the body are extremely complex; they involve multiple interrelationships among autogenous biochemicals, exogenous drugs, foods, and other environmental substances.
2 ☐ Hormone imbalances tend to be multiple; because of the interrelatedness of the endocrine glands, alteration of levels of one hormone often cause secondary changes in levels of other hormones.
3 ☐ Hormones are extremely potent chemicals: dosages of pure hormones are often measured in microgram doses.
4 ☐ Bioassay techniques allow accurate administration of doses measured in units, even when the drugs are not refined or when their active ingredients are unknown.
5 ☐ Changing the molecular structure of a hormone drug can increase its selectivity but side effects cannot be eliminated completely.
6 ☐ Successful therapy with hormones and hormone antagonists requires careful and continuous monitoring of hormone balance and response to the drugs.
7 ☐ Active participation by clients in their therapeutic regimens is critical for the management of chronic conditions involving hormone therapy.
8 ☐ Use of hormones and hormone antagonists tends to require therapy over a long period of time—often for life.
9 ☐ Physical dependence on hormones may occur when hormone drugs trigger negative feedback systems controlling endocrine function and cause atrophy of secreting glands; when this occurs, clients must be withdrawn gradually (weaned) from drug regimens.
10 ☐ Timing of drug doses is critical to effective therapy (*e.g.*, administration of replacement hormones, synchronization of hormone therapy with the reproductive cycle).
11 ☐ Hormone imbalances tend to be insidious in onset. Toxicity to hormone and hormone antagonists also develops insidiously. Assessment skills of the nurse are critical to early detection of problems.
12 ☐ Pronounced hormone imbalances produce medical crises that are life-threatening.
13 ☐ Genetic engineering techniques may provide more plentiful supplies of human-specific hormones with reduced antigenic potential.
14 ☐ Protein hormones must be carefully stored and handled to prevent deterioration.
15 ☐ Hormone drugs are often marketed as depot preparations that are absorbed slowly.
16 ☐ Special precautions are required to safeguard persons exposed to radioactive medications.
17 ☐ Tracer doses of radionuclides impose minimal radiation risk, whereas therapeutic doses emit toxic doses of ionizing radiation.
18 ☐ Radioactivity of radionuclides decreases exponentially with the passage of time; radioactive half-life ($t_{1/2}$) equals the length of time required for the radioactivity of a substance to decline by 50%.
19 ☐ Rapid progress in pharmaceutic research and development makes continuing study critical to safe use of drug substances in the future.

Teaching Strategies

Chapter 34 may be assigned to students along with Chapters 32, 33, 36 and the portion of Chapter 22 that deals with hormones produced by the sympathetic nervous system and adrenal medulla.

1 ☐ Students should be directed to review the anatomy and physiology of the thyroid, parathyroid, and pituitary glands before and during the study of this chapter.
2 ☐ Because of the complexity of the endocrine system, it is difficult to organize the progression of learning from the simple to the complex. Early class discussions could center on hormones such as

parathormone, however, because their control mechanisms do not appear to involve the pituitary tropic hormones.

Evaluation Examples (Test Item)

ESSAY QUESTION

1. Discuss briefly the role of the pituitary in the control of glucocorticoid and thyroid hormone production.

MULTIPLE CHOICE ITEMS

1. For which of the following hormones is the timing of replacement doses most critical?

1. Thyroid hormone
2. Vasopressin
3. ACTH

*4. Insulin

2. For which of the following hormones is the timing of replacement doses least important?

*1. Thyroid hormone

2. Glucocorticoids
3. Topical estrogens
4. Oral contraceptives

UNIT NINE: DRUGS AFFECTING SPECIFIC BODY SYSTEMS

35
Drugs Affecting the Respiratory Tract

Chapter 35 describes basic nursing actions for clients receiving drug therapy to facilitate respiratory functions. In particular, it addresses pharmacologic treatment and nursing management required for clients with airway obstructions caused by bronchitis, emphysema, and asthma. An assumption is made that the nursing student has already completed courses in anatomy, physiology, health assessment, and nursing fundamentals (or basic comfort measures). This chapter does not discuss all the medication used to treat respiratory disorders (drugs such as antibiotics, cold remedies, antihistamines, decongestants, corticosteroids, narcotics, muscle relaxants, and respiratory stimulants are covered in other chapters). Instead, this chapter deals with specific drugs and treatment or nursing measures for clients with respiratory disturbances as a result of bronchitis, emphysema, and asthma.

The text begins with a brief description of the basic physiology of bronchoconstriction and bronchodilation, followed by a discussion of the etiology and pathology of asthma, bronchitis, and emphysema. This helps the student to understand the mode of action and desired therapeutic effects on pharmacologic therapy directed at promoting bronchodilation. Other drugs that support respiratory effort, methods of delivering oxygen, and inhalation therapy, and nursing management aimed at promoting respiratory function, are addressed. Through the study of this chapter, the student may develop the following concepts:

1 □ Nursing has a vital role in respiratory care.
2 □ Respiratory disease produces anxiety in clients and their families, and perhaps in the nursing student.
3 □ Emergency situations arise that require prompt action and treatment to establish and maintain a patient airway.
4 □ Environmental and etiologic factors contribute to respiratory compromise.
5 □ Treatment is directed at the following:
- **a.** Decreasing airway resistance
- **b.** Relieving bronchospasm
- **c.** Providing bronchodilation
- **d.** Promoting hydration
- **e.** Providing humidification
- **f.** Decreasing the viscosity and amount of secretions
- **g.** Removing secretions

6 □ Clients can be assisted to live productive and meaningful lives.

Teaching Strategies

1 □ Students may define or discuss the following:
- **a.** Respiration and normal anatomy and physiology of the respiratory system. Include normal control of respiration, mechanism of pulmonary ventilation, and gas exchange. Describe internal and external factors that affect the respiratory system.
- **b.** Sympathetic and parasympathetic nervous system
- **c.** Immune system
- **d.** Bronchoconstriction and bronchodilation
- **e.** Respiratory failure; pathophysiology of asthma, bronchitis, and emphysema
- **f.** Signs and symptoms of decreased oxygen and of increased carbon dioxide levels

2 □ Arrange for students to analyze a series of blood gas results.
3 □ Students may complete drug cards for the pharmacologic agents.
4 □ Students may develop a patient care plan for clients with asthma, bronchitis, and emphysema, including the teaching component.
5 □ Have students observe films on assessment of the chest and have them listen to tapes of breath sounds. They may practice on each other. Students should care for clients with chest pathology, and then review laboratory and x-ray results. Students should

listen to the chest before and after respiratory therapy.

6 □ Arrange for students to observe clients undergoing pulmonary function tests. Guide discussions of the results. Compare and contrast them to normal values. Students may try pulmonary function tests and compare their values to those of patients.

7 □ If possible, arrange for students to try out an IPPB machine, aerosol-nebulizer, or inhaler on themselves. They may discuss what they felt. Students may instruct each other on how to use and care for the equipment.

8 □ Break the class up into groups of students. Present a case study of a client with advanced pulmonary emphysema. Give each group an assignment related to an aspect of the care of the client, and have each group report back to the whole class. Topics might include the following: rationale and technique of coughing and deep breathing; nursing actions to mobilize and remove secretions; factors affecting learning in respiratory clients and important points to include in client education; drug interactions; and nutritional aspects.

9 □ The following are examples of audiovisual materials:

a. From Trainex: Acid-Base Balance: 994—Patient Assessment; 996—Management of Respiratory Acidosis and Alkalosis. Human Anatomy and Physiology (Dr. Muzio's cassettes): 17—Respiration; Oxygen Administration

b. From J.B. Lippincott Company, Lippincott Learning System (filmstrip, manual, cassette): Respiratory Care: Concepts and Techniques; Deep Breathing and Coughing; Nasotracheal Suctioning: Cuff and Cannula; Tracheostomy Care—Principles; Tracheostomy Care—Practice; Mechanical Intervention; Oxygen Therapy—Principles; Oxygen Therapy—Practice

c. From J.B. Lippincott Company: Bates B: A Visual Guide to Physical Examination, 2nd ed, Thorax and Lung

d. From Humetrics Corp.: Chest Signs–Sounds

Evaluation Examples (Test Items)

MULTIPLE CHOICE ITEMS

1. Mr. LH, with chronic obstructive lung disease (advanced emphysema), receives Mucomyst through an IPPB machine every 4 hours when awake. This has been prescribed to

1. Stimulate coughing
2. Dilate the bronchial tree
3. "Wet" the secretions
*4. Liquefy bronchial secretions

2. In supplying oxygen to LH, who has a low PO_2 and a high PCO_2, the method of choice for delivery is by

1. Nasal catheter
2. Oxygen tent
*3. Venturi mask
4. Positive pressure mask

3. Pulmonary agents by IPPB machine are ordered for LH. You should administer these medications in which order?

*1. Wetting agent, bronchodilator, mycolytic agent, antibiotic
2. Mucolytic agent, bronchodilator, antibiotic, vasoconstrictor
3. Vasoconstrictor, wetting agent, mucolytic agent, antibiotic
4. Wetting agent, mucolytic agent, bronchodilator, antibiotic

4. The purpose of percussion and vibration is to

1. Stimulate a patient to cough
*2. Loosen secretions
3. Open the airway initially
4. Prevent atelectasis

5. LH is receiving low-flow oxygen, and while administering morning care you note that his conjunctivae are red. Your nursing actions should include

a. Washing his eyes with saline solution
b. Stopping the oxygen
c. Checking vital signs
d. Continuing the oxygen
e. Checking the oxygen administration set-up for humidity

1. a, b, d, e
*2. a, d, e
3. b, c
4. d only

6. Mrs. RS is on a ß-receptor stimulator drug for bronchodilation. Which of the following effects would you *not* expect to find?

1. Nervousness
2. Increased demand for oxygen by the heart
*3. Bradycardia
4. Precordial distress and pounding in the chest

7. In the hospital, Mrs. BT is receiving Isuprel. Nursing actions would include monitoring her

a. Pulse
b. Blood pressure
c. Level of consciousness
d. ECG

1. a, b
*2. a, b, d
3. b only
4. All of the above

8. BT has just been placed on aminophylline. Nursing actions would include

a. Assessing the patient for nausea and restlessness
b. Checking the chart for BT's drug level
c. Asking BT if she smokes
d. Checking to see if BT has a history of gastrointestinal bleeding

1. a only
2. a, c, d
3. b, d
*4. All of the above

9. Mr. WL, a hospitalized patient, has been diagnosed as having asthma. Which of the following drugs would you *not* expect him to be on?

1. Aminophylline
2. Vanceril
*3. Aspirin
4. Cromolyn sodium

10. Mr. TS, with long-standing chronic obstructive pulmonary disease, has been admitted with left lower lobe pneumonia. His *p*H is 7.02, PO_2 is 42, and PCO_2 is 98. He has been intubated and placed on a respirator delivering 60% oxygen to maintain normal blood gas levels. After a few days lung compliance continues to decrease, and respiratory failure progresses. The most likely reason for this is

*1. Oxygen toxicity
2. Advancing emphysema
3. Superimposed infection
4. Inadequate dose of bronchodilators

36
Drugs Affecting the Reproductive Systems and Sexuality

Reproductive Systems
Physiology and Hormones of the Reproductive Systems
Drugs and the Reproductive Systems
Nursing Management
Sexuality and Sexual Behavior
Sexually Transmitted Diseases
Drugs Affecting Sexual Behavior
Drugs Used in Treatment of Sexual Problems
Nursing Management
Contraceptives
Male Contraceptive Measures
Female Contraceptive Measures
Nursing Management
Infertility and Fertility Drugs
Male Infertility
Female Infertility
Nursing Management

Chapter 36 presents material on the effects of a wide variety of substances on sexual response and fertility, as well as the growth and development of the reproductive system.

Estrogens and androgens are present in differing levels in both men and women. The balance of the two affect performance and secondary sexual characteristics. Shifts in their levels occur at the menarche, during pregnancy and lactation, and at menopause in women, and during puberty and climacteric in men. In some instances, medical manipulation of hormone levels may be needed to treat certain conditions.

Both men and women may practice fertility control. Various methods of contraception are discussed briefly in this chapter. Treatments for infertility and the effects of various drugs on libido are also presented.

Students responsible for giving medication in any setting benefit from a review of this chapter. The student can be assisted to develop the following concepts:

1 □ The effects of some medications on sexual interest and functioning can be anticipated.
2 □ Psychotropic drugs and mood regulators have specific effects on sexual response and function.
3 □ The nurse should be knowledgeable about menopause and estrogen replacement therapy, as well as ovulatory stimulation for infertility.
4 □ Various methods of contraception are available to men and women, and each has benefits and disadvantages that must be taken into consideration when discussing methods with a client.
5 □ Condoms are used for protection against sexually transmitted diseases as well as for contraception.

Teaching Strategies

1 □ Classroom discussion may benefit from consideration of the following:
  a. Discuss the various contraceptive measures available to men and women. Include religious considerations as well as information on efficacy and safety.
  b. Discuss the effects of alcohol, marijuana, and cocaine on male sexual function.
2 □ The part of Chapter 32 that deals with male and female sex hormones may be combined with this chapter for additional reading and discussion.
3 □ Discuss the effect of noncompliance on the effectiveness of oral contraceptives.
4 □ Have contraceptive methods on display.
5 □ A representative from a local women's group may speak to the class on contraception and on her experiences in local health-care agencies. Alternatively, students may visit an agency or clinic offering contraceptive services.
6 □ A nurse or health-care provider from a sex therapy clinic may be invited to speak to the class about the effects of certain drugs on libido.

Evaluation Examples (Test Items)

ESSAY QUESTIONS

1. Explain the ways in which anticholinergic and antiadrenergic drugs affect sexual activity.

2. Why is a complete history of current drug use necessary when patients complain of impairment of sexual functioning?

3. Discuss the relationship of dietary deficiencies and exercise to amenorrhea, female infertility, and to menopause.

4. Discuss estrogen replacement therapy during the menopause. Identify comfort measures that are alternatives to medication.

5. Discuss three protective measures that should be employed by health-care providers caring for patients who may have AIDS.

MULTIPLE CHOICE ITEMS

1. Premenstrual syndrome is manifested by
  a. Mood swings
  b. Fluid retention
  c. Migraine-type headaches

d. A decrease in progesterone level
1. a, c
2. b, d
3. c, e
4. d, e
*5. All of the above

2. Dysmenorrhea can be treated by medications that
1. Increase prostaglandin production
*2. Inhibit prostaglandin production
3. Increase progesterone production
4. Inhibit progesterone production

37 Drugs Affecting the Musculoskeletal System: Skeletal Muscle Relaxants and Antispastic Agents

Chapter 37 briefly discusses the physiology of muscle contraction and the pathophysiology of peripheral muscle spasms and spasticity from central nervous system damage. It discusses drugs used to relax skeletal muscles and treat spasticity.

Through the study of this chapter, students may develop the following concepts:

1 □ Skeletal muscle relaxants are used to relieve the pain and to increase the mobility of affected muscles in acute musculoskeletal disorders.
2 □ In some situations it cannot be determined whether the benefits of a given drug in this group of drugs come primarily from its muscle-relaxing properties or from its sedative effect.
3 □ There is no completely satisfactory form of therapy for alleviating skeletal muscle spasticity.
4 □ Skeletal muscle relaxants cause drowsiness and dizziness as adverse reactions, and clients should exercise caution in operating vehicles and machinery when using these drugs.

Teaching Strategies

□ Classroom discussion may be stimulated by consideration of questions such as the following:

a. How would you assess a client for beneficial response to a skeletal muscle relaxant? If the client has had severe muscle spasms, what activities of daily living might be accomplished more easily if the skeletal muscle relaxant is of benefit?
b. What types of adverse reactions occur with skeletal muscle relaxants? Name specific drugs and give an example of an adverse reaction for each.
c. When might a skeletal muscle relaxant not be warranted (when spasticity actually contributed to ambulation efforts)?

Evaluation Examples (Test Items)

MULTIPLE CHOICE ITEMS

1. The most common adverse reactions with skeletal muscle relaxants are
*1. Drowsiness and dizziness
2. Impaired renal and liver functions
3. Arrhythmias and shortness of breath
4. Hypersensitivity reactions and anaphylaxis

2. An example of a benzodiazepine that is used as a skeletal muscle relaxant is
1. Acetylsalicylic acid
2. Carisoprodol
*3. Valium
4. Orphenadrine

3. A skeletal muscle relaxant that must not be given to the client receiving a monoamine oxidase (MAO) inhibitor is
1. Carisoprodol
*2. Cyclobenzaprine
3. Valium
4. Baclofen

4. A skeletal muscle relaxant that may work by decreasing the amount of calcium released within muscle fibers is
1. Cyclobenzaprine
*2. Dantrolene
3. Baclofen
4. Valium

5. Many paraplegics have been helped in particular by
1. Cyclobenzaprine
*2. Dantrolene
3. Baclofen
4. Valium

6. A useful medication for clients with nocturnal leg cramps is
1. Cyclobenzaprine
2. Baclofen
*3. Quinine
4. Carisoprodol

38 Drugs Affecting the Kidneys: Diuretics

Chapter 38 discusses kidney physiology, pathologic conditions involving fluid retention and tissue edema, and drugs administered to promote the elimination of fluids through the kidneys.

Through the study of this chapter, students may develop the following concepts:

1 □ Chemical agents can alter physiologic processes in the kidneys and influence the excretion of salts and water.
2 □ Diuresis initiates a positive feedback mechanism whereby increased flow rates in the tubule reduce electrolyte reabsorption, further increasing fluid excretion and flow rates.
3 □ Potassium imbalance is a frequent complication of diuretic therapy; both deficiencies and excesses can occur, depending on the specific drugs employed.
4 □ Manifestations of diuretic toxicity may include deficiency of all electrolytes, dehydration, and acid-base imbalance.
5 □ Diuretic toxicity is more likely to develop in clients who are under stress, particularly those exposed to a warm humid environment.
6 □ It is important that health professionals (physicians, nurses, and pharmacists) be fully informed about treatment, particularly the drugs, a client is taking.
7 □ Several diuretics increase the severity of gout and diabetes mellitus.
8 □ Osmotic diuretics exert a biphasic effect on blood volume, initially increasing it and subsequently decreasing it when diuresis has been established.
9 □ Adverse reactions to drugs may be minimized by the concurrent use of two or more drugs with opposite side effects (*e.g.,* potassium-wasting and potassium-sparing diuretics).
10 □ Diuretics are best administered in the morning so that maximum diuretic effect is exerted during the waking hours.
11 □ When drugs are given that alter a body function, nursing care must be adjusted to meet the changed needs of the client.
12 □ Fluid, electrolyte, and acid-base balances are complex and interrelated; drug therapy that alters one part of the system influences many other parts as well.
13 □ Response to drug therapy is influenced by multiple factors, including diet, environmental conditions, emotional reactions, and stress.
14 □ A given physiologic effect (such as diuresis) may be the therapeutic goal of one treatment regimen (diuretic therapy) but a side effect of another (xanthine therapy in obstructive lung disease).

Teaching Strategies

1 □ A sound knowledge of fluid and electrolyte homeostasis is essential for students to understand the action of diuretics. The study of these drugs should begin with a review of the anatomy and physiology of the kidney and the body's fluid, electrolyte, and acid-base balances. If students have not been exposed to material on pathologic states involving imbalances in these systems, this aspect of pathophysiology should be introduced. Students should also review nutrition relating to foods that influence fluid, electrolyte, and acid-base balances. The study of this chapter may profitably be integrated with Chapters 27, 28, and 29 in a unit on cardiovascular disease.
2 □ Students involved in clinical practice with clients should monitor the fluid, electrolyte, and acid-base balances of all their clients. Data from the clients' histories, physical examinations, and laboratory findings should be related to factors influencing the clients' fluid, electrolyte, and acid-base balances. If diuretics have been administered, sequential data that would indicate client response to the medications should be reviewed.
3 □ Response to stress markedly influences chemical balance and response to diuretic therapy in clients receiving these drugs. Diuretic therapy is a good example of a medication regimen whose efficacy is altered by multiple factors, including other drugs, disease, diet, environmental influences, and coping strategies for managing stress.
4 □ Students may develop a teaching plan for assisting a client to avoid fluid, electrolyte, and acid-base imbalances while on a drug regimen that includes prescriptions of digoxin and chlorothiazide.
5 □ With the assistance of tables listing the nutritional content of foods, students may prepare a list of foods that are high in potassium and low in sodium, noting which of these also provide ample quantities of magnesium and calcium. The following may be discussed: (*a*) factors influencing acceptability of these foods by clients who need potassium-rich diets; and

(*b*) pharmacologic effects of these foods, such as nervous system stimulation, that might limit the quantity that can be used by the client.

Evaluation Examples (Test Items)

ESSAY QUESTIONS

1. Compare and contrast the mechanisms of action of mannitol, chlorothiazide (Diuril), acetazolamide (Diamox), and spironolactone (Aldactone). Indicate which of these diuretics are potassium-wasting and which are potassium-sparing.

2. Discuss fluid and electrolyte problems likely to occur in clients receiving digitalis and diuretics simultaneously. Describe two or more nursing measures for preventing or ameliorating these problems.

TRUE AND FALSE STATEMENTS

_F_ **1.** Cardiac arrest caused by hypokalemia responds well to cardiopulmonary resuscitation.

_T_ **2.** Diuresis tends to promote more diuresis.

_T_ **3.** The abdominal symptoms caused by hypokalemia in clients who are also receiving digitalis are apt to differ from those of clients not receiving digitalis.

_F_ **4.** Symptoms of hyperkalemia include intestinal atony.

_F_ **5.** Diuretics are most apt to cause toxic symptoms during cold damp weather.

_T_ **6.** Diuretics are most apt to cause serious hypokalemia in clients experiencing high levels of stress.

_F_ **7.** Most fruit juices contain high levels of potassium.

_F_ **8.** Diuretics are often prescribed for the treatment of anuria.

_F_ **9.** Carbonic anhydrase inhibitors are often administered prior to eye surgery for their diuretic effects.

MULTIPLE CHOICE ITEMS

1. Which of the following diuretics loses effectiveness when administered over a long period of time?
  1. Mannitol
  2. Chlorothiazide
  3. Spironolactone
  *4 Ammonium chloride

2. Signs and symptoms of hypokalemia secondary to diuresis include
  a. Abdominal distention and constipation
  b. Signs and symptoms of digitalis toxicity in clients taking digitalis
  c. A tendency toward tetany
  *1. a, b
  2. a, c
  3. b, c
  4. All of the above

3. A diuretic used to reduce intraocular pressure is
  1. Furosemide
  2. Spironolactone
  3. Chlorothiazide
  *4. Glycerol

4. The action of most diuretics can be enhanced by limiting dietary intake of
  1. Water
  *2. Sodium
  3. Potassium
  4. Calcium

5. To reduce undesirable side effects of diuretics, it is important to maintain proper levels of
  1. Calcium
  *2. Potassium
  3. Vitamin A
  4. Vitamin C

6. Which of the following are potassium-sparing diuretics?
  a. Furosemide
  b. Spironolactone
  c. Chlorothiazide
  d. Mannitol
  1. a, b
  2. a, c
  *3. b only
  4. c, d
  5. d only

7. Which of the following supplies significant amounts of potassium?
  1. Apple juice
  2. Cranberry juice
  3. Ginger ale
  *4. Orange juice

SITUATION-BASED MULTIPLE CHOICE ITEMS

Situation: Ms. RG, age 61 years, is to have surgery for cataracts. She is to receive glycerin preoperatively the morning of surgery.

1. The glycerin is most likely to be administered
  *1. Orally, despite the fact that RG is to have surgery
  2. Parenterally, because she will be NPO before surgery
  3. Intravenously, in the operating room
  4. Topically, to the eye

2. Initial reactions to the glycerin are likely to include
  1. Slight nausea and a drop in blood pressure
  *2. Slight nausea and a rise in blood pressure
  3. Intestinal cramping and a drop in blood pressure
  4. Intestinal cramping and a rise in blood pressure

3. The glycerin is administered to
   1. Prevent hypovolemic shock during surgery
   2. Prevent hypertension from stress response during surgery
   3. Promote vascular flow to the cornea of the eye
   *4. Reduce intraocular pressure

4. In this case, the diuresis that follows administration of glycerin would be
   1. A therapeutic response
   *2. A side effect
   3. A toxic effect
   4. Somewhat risky, in view of RG's age

5. Because RG has received glycerin, her postoperative blood pressure would be
   1. Higher than it would be otherwise
   *2. Lower than it would be otherwise
   3. Erratic, fluctuating from high to low
   4. Unaffected

6. What happens to the glycerin that is absorbed systemically?
   1. All of it is metabolized for energy
   2. All of it is excreted through the kidneys
   *3. Some of it is metabolized for energy and some of it is excreted through the kidneys
   4. It is metabolized by the liver and excreted through the bile

Situation: Mr. SL, age 70 years, has responded well to treatment for congestive heart failure. He is found to have hypertension (blood pressure range of 180/200-100/110), and hydrochlorothiazide has been prescribed.

1. Before SL begins taking hydrochlorothiazide, he should be assessed for
   a. Electrolytes, especially sodium and potassium
   b. Glucose and history of diabetes mellitus
   c. Uric acid and a history of gout
   1. a, b
   2. a, c
   3. b, c
   *4. All of the above

2. The diuretic is likely to be administered
   *1. Orally
   2. Subcutaneously
   3. Intramuscularly
   4. Intravenously

3. At what time of day should the medication be taken?
   1. At bedtime
   2. With meals, three times a day
   *3. As early in the day as possible
   4. At any time, provided it is given at the same time of day every day

4. SL should be monitored regularly for
   a. Vital signs
   b. Muscle spasms
   c. Serum concentrations of potassium
   d. Hyperglycemia
   1. a, b, c
   2. a, b, d
   *3. a, c, d
   4. b, c, d
   5. All of the above

5. SL should be taught to report to the nurse or physician
   *1. Feelings of weakness and malaise
   2. Pounding headaches
   3. Marked hunger between meals
   4. Unusually large outputs of urine

UNIT TEN: DRUGS USED FOR NEOPLASTIC DISEASE

39 Theoretic Base for Chemotherapy, Alkylating Agents, and Antimetabolites

Physiology of Cells: The Cell Cycle
Pathophysiology of Cells: Cancer
The Use of Antineoplastic Drugs
Factors in Making Decisions
Cell Growth
Type of Malignancy
Pharmacologic Factors
Physiologic Status
Previous Antineoplastic Drug Therapy
Alkylating Agents
Nitrogen Mustards
Mechlorethamine
Cyclophosphamide
Melphalan or L-Sarcolysin
Chlorambucil
Ethylenimines and Methylmelamines
Alkysulfonate
Busulfan
Nitrosoureas
Carmustine
Lomustine
Streptozocin
Triazene
Dacarbazine
Platinum Complex
Cisplatin
Piperzine Derivative
Pipobroman
Antimetabolites
Folic Acid Analogue
Methotrexate
Pyrimidine Analogues
Fluorouracil and Floxuridine
Cytarabine
Purine Analogues
Mercaptopurine
Thioguanine
Nursing Management
Nursing Implications
Nursing Process
Assessment
Diagnosis
Planning
Interventions
Client Education
Evaluation

Chapter 39 begins by briefly discussing the physiology of the various phases of the cell cycle. This is to assist the student in understanding the concept of cycle-dependent and cycle-independent antineoplastic drugs. General aspects of antineoplastic drug therapy are briefly discussed. These general aspects include remission, first-order kinetics, dosage determination, and toxicity.

Several factors are discussed that affect whether or not antineoplastic drug therapy is used for a client's cancer, and, if so, what specific agents are selected.

Through the study of this chapter, students may develop the following concepts:

1 □ Complete remission of a neoplastic condition does not mean cure.
2 □ Antineoplastic drugs do not kill every tumor cell; rather, they kill a certain percentage of cells.
3 □ Outcomes with several cancers, such as acute lymphocytic leukemia, have been significantly improved through the use of combination therapy.
4 □ Blood levels of antineoplastic drug correlate better with drug dosage on the basis of body surface area than on the basis of milligrams per kilogram.
5 □ Cycle-independent drugs work during all phases of the cell's mitotic cycle and cycle-dependent drugs work only during certain phases of the cycle.
6 □ Solid tumors often have a large percentage of their cell mass in the G_0 phase of the cell cycle. Cells in this phase are not sensitive to many antineoplastic drugs.
7 □ Tumors that have a large percentage of their cells actively synthesizing DNA and dividing during a short time span are more susceptible to antineoplastic drug action.
8 □ Most antineoplastic drugs are relatively insoluble in lipids; access to the brain is limited to molecules that are fat-soluble.
9 □ The client's overall status affects the use of antineoplastic therapy because, as status declines, the ability to tolerate normal doses of antineoplastic drugs generally declines as well.
10 □ Cancer cells develop resistance to drugs by more than one mechanism.
11 □ Several complications apply to many of the antineoplastic agents (anorexia, taste changes, nausea, and vomiting; stomatitis; bone marrow suppression, including anemia, leukopenia, and thrombocytopenia;

and alopecia), and all nurses dealing with these drugs should be well versed in the nursing interventions that relate to these common complications.

Teaching Strategies

□ Classroom discussion may be stimulated by consideration of questions such as the following:

a. What are the four major complications of antineoplastic drug therapy? Discuss nursing interventions relative to each of these major complications.

b. Define what is meant by complete remission. Describe how you would explain the term and its ramifications to your client.

c. Identify the factors that determine whether antineoplastic drug therapy is used for a client's cancer.

Evaluation Examples (Test Items)

ESSAY QUESTIONS

1. Explain the various phases of the cell cycle.

2. Select one of the four major complications of antineoplastic drug therapy. Describe nursing interventions that could be used when your client experiences this complication.

3. Explain the usual precautions taken when an antineoplastic drug is a vesicant and must be administered intravenously.

4. Explain the usual interventions taken when an antineoplastic drug causes hyperuricemia and hyperuricosuria.

MULTIPLE CHOICE ITEMS

1. Mechlorethamine is an example of which type of alkylating agent?

*1. Nitrogen mustard
2. Ethylenimine derivative
3. Alkylsulfonate
4. Nitrosourea
5. Triazene

2. The most commonly used antineoplastic drug is

1. Thioguanine
2. Mechlorethamine
*3. Cyclophosphamide
4. Carmustine
5. Chlorambucil

3. Hemorrhagic cystitis and bladder malignancy are complications that can occur with the use of

1. Fluorouracil
2. Mercaptopurine
3. Busulfan
*4. Cyclophosphamide
5. Chlorambucil

4. The only alkylating agents to cross the blood–brain barrier are

1. Nitrogen mustards
2. Ethylenimines
3. Alkylsulfonates
*4. Nitrosoureas
5. Triazenes

5. Methotrexate is used for

1. Remission induction in acute lymphocytic leukemia
*2. Maintenance of remissions in acute lymphocytic leukemia
3. Management of cancer of the esophagus
4. Treatment of cancer of the pancreas

6. Mercaptopurine is an example of

1. Folic acid analogue
2. Pyrimidine analogue
*3. Purine analogue
4. Alkylating agent

40
Natural Products, Hormones, and Miscellaneous Agents

Natural Products
Plant Alkaloids: Vinca Alkaloids
Vinblastine
Vincristine
Other Plant Alkaloids
Etoposide
Antibiotics
Bleomycin
Dactinomycin
Daunorubicin
Doxorubicin
Mitomycin
Plicamycin
Enzyme
Asparaginase
Hormones
Adrenocorticosteroids
Estrogens and Androgens
Progestins
Antiestrogen
Tamoxifen
Synthetic Estrogen Antimetabolite
Estramustine Phosphate
Miscellaneous Agents
Hydroxyurea
Mitotane
Procarbazine
Aminoglutethimide
Nursing Management
Nursing Process

Chapter 40 is a continuation of Chapter 39 in that the general concepts covered in Chapter 39 apply to the specific antineoplastic agents discussed in Chapter 40.

Through the study of this chapter, students may develop the following concepts:

1 □ Some potent antineoplastic agents have their origins in plants known about for hundreds of years (periwinkle and mandrake plants).
2 □ Several antibiotics, natural products of certain microorganisms, have use as antineoplastic agents.
3 □ The management of some cancers can involve the concept of nutritional deprivation of the cancer.
4 □ It is possible to change the course of the neoplastic process in some tissues to some degree by changing the hormonal environment of such tumors.
5 □ The treatment of a cancer with antineoplastic agents may be related to the subsequent development of a second cancer in the treated individual.
6 □ Several complications apply to many of the antineoplastic agents (anorexia, nausea, and vomiting; bone marrow suppression; alopecia), and all nurses dealing with these drugs should be well versed in the related nursing interventions.

Teaching Strategies

□ Classroom discussion may be stimulated by consideration of questions such as the following:

a. Discuss the role of estrogens and androgens with cancer. What is the rationale for their use? When would estrogens be used in women? Why would male clients be treated with hormones?
b. The current treatment of choice for testicular cancer involves two antineoplastic agents studied in this chapter. The MOPP regimen for Hodgkin's Disease utilizes three agents studied in this chapter. Discuss the nurse's role in early detection of these cancers.
c. Explain the syndrome of inappropriate secretion of antidiuretic hormone and what assessment observations the nurse should make.

Evaluation Examples (Test Items)

ESSAY QUESTIONS

1. Select one of the four major complications of antineoplastic drug therapy. Describe nursing interventions that could be used when your client experiences this complication.

2. Describe the neurotoxicities that may occur when vincristine is used and identify appropriate interventions for the client experiencing these toxicities.

3. Describe the mechanism of action of antibiotics as antineoplastic agents.

4. Explain different roles the adrenocorticosteroids may play in the management of various cancers.

MULTIPLE CHOICE ITEMS

1. An example of a drug that causes alopecia is
1. Vinblastine
2. Prednisone
*3. Dactinomycin
4. Tamoxifen

2. An unusual feature of vincristine, as an antineoplastic agent, is that it is
1. Given intravenously
2. Administered on a weekly basis

3. An agent that causes alopecia
*4. A bone marrow-sparing agent

3. Bleomycin causes a toxic reaction in lung tissue progressing from a pneumonitis to a pulmonary fibrosis. This is because

1. The drug is used with squamous cell carcinoma of the lung
*2. Lungs do not have the enzyme bleohydrolase
3. Older men are frequently the recipients of this drug
4. The drug disrupts the DNA molecule's repair mechanism

4. A major use of dactinomycin is in the treatment of

*1. Wilms' tumor
2. Cancer of the pancreas
3. Acute lymphocytic leukemia
4. Cancer of the esophagus

5. A drug important in the treatment of hypercalcemia and hypercalciuria secondary to metastatic disease is

1. Bleomycin
2. Daunorubicin
3. Dactinomycin
*4. Plicamycin

UNIT ELEVEN: DRUGS AFFECTING THE IMMUNE SYSTEM

41 Drugs Used in the Treatment of Allergy

Pathophysiology of Allergies
Allergens, Manifestations, and Intervention
Urticaria and Angioedema
Atopic Dermatitis and Eczema
Noneczematous Dermatitis
Drug Reactions
Insect Bites
Nasal Hypersensitivity
Allergic Rhinitis
Allergic Ocular Disorders
Bronchial Asthma
Hypersensitivity Pneumonitis
Testing for Allergies
Skin Testing
Other Tests
Nursing Management
Nursing Implications

Chapter 41 considers the effects of various substances that may result in allergic reactions. The importance of accurate nursing observations and history taking is stressed because these narrow the list of possible allergens and may decrease the need for extensive testing.

Allergic reactions vary from mild discomforts that are easily treated by substance avoidance or medication to life-threatening situations that require hospitalization. Treatment may have to be instituted immediately to save the client's life.

It is estimated that 5% of clients require hospitalization because of drug reactions, and that 10% of hospitalized clients experience at least one adverse drug reaction. These statistics emphasize the need for accurate reporting by nurses, including descriptions of urticaria, angioedema, gastrointestinal or vascular symptoms, nasal hypersensitivity, asthma, generalized autoimmune-type body reactions, and episodes of respiratory or cardiac difficulties.

The use of intradermal or prick tests, or of immunoglobulin serum levels to establish a correct diagnosis, require nursing preparation of the client as well as proper storage and usage of the testing materials. Treatment includes client education about the removal of offending substances whenever possible, and about the appropriate use of specific medications.

Through the study of this chapter, the student should be assisted in developing the following concepts:

1 □ The nurse should be familiar with all types of allergic reactions–the signs, the symptoms, and how they progress.
2 □ Professional nurses should appreciate the importance of accurate observations and histories relating to allergies.
3 □ No drugs should be regarded as totally without danger.
4 □ Reactions may result in external or internal manifestations that are acute or chronic, which may appear immediately on contact with the allergen or not until a week or more has passed.

Teaching Strategies

1 □ After students complete the table in the workbook, they may discuss it in class or in small groups.
2 □ Have the students interview five hospitalized patients for histories of prehospitalization allergies, and for evidence of any allergies caused by substances used since admission. Have them report back to the class.
3 □ Have the students draw up a teaching protocol to be used with all patients who are to undergo prick or intradermal skin tests. Under supervision they may use their teaching strategies on patients about to undergo these allergy tests.
4 □ Have the students interview five patients for common over-the-counter drugs used for self-medication. Analyze at least three of these for ingredients that may conflict with those in prescription medications they are taking.

Evaluation Examples (Test Items)

ESSAY QUESTIONS

1. Describe the sequence of an allergic reaction.
2. Discuss the use of ß-adrenergic drugs in the treatment of some type 1 sensitivities.
3. Describe three different medication regimens commonly used for the treatment of bronchial asthma.
4. Name three common reactions to antihistamine therapy, with the appropriate treatments, that should be incorporated into client education.
5. List three important factors to be stressed with patients requiring steroid therapy.

42 Drugs Used for Immunity

Chapter 42 presents material on immunity and immunizing agents. Active and passive acquired immunities are discussed, along with programs for, and opinions about, immunization. The actions of vaccines and toxoids are explained, as well as possible reactions to their use.

It is important for students to understand how the immune response is elicited, because it is the body's third line of defense against microorganisms. Immunoglobulins, the protective antibodies, are needed to fight infectious agents (antigens) that enter the body. This protection is offered by an immunoglobulin found in the colostrum of lactating women, as well as in gamma globulin, vaccines, and toxoids.

Vaccinations are not given without some risks. Those who are allergic may have responses that vary from minor discomfort to anaphylactic shock. In addition, some illnesses have been linked to the administration of vaccines. A prime example of this is the number of people who developed Guillain-Barré syndrome after receiving injections to protect them against swine flu in 1976.

Reevaluation of vaccination programs is ongoing. Within the past few years, routine smallpox vaccinations have been discontinued in most areas of the world, while others (HBV, VZIG) have been instituted.

Students should find this chapter helpful in gaining an understanding of the mechanisms of immunity. The following concepts may be developed:

1 □ The professional nurse should be aware of the ways in which antigen-antibody responses take place.
2 □ There are various types of immunity.
3 □ There are immune systems disorders, and they may be primary or secondary.
4 □ The professional nurse should be knowledgeable about programs for immunization, including schedules, methods, and dosages.
5 □ The professional nurse should be aware of the use of monoclonal antibodies to strengthen the immune system and prevent transplant rejection.

Teaching Strategies

1 □ Classroom discussion may be stimulated by the following types of questions:
- **a.** A vaccine for hepatitis B (serum hepatitis) is now available. Discuss any advantages or disadvantages of offering this vaccine to health-care providers.
- **b.** What information can be given to parents who question the wisdom of routine immunization of children against pertussis?
- **c.** What steps should be taken to be certain that a vaccine is safe for use?
- **d.** Discuss natural immunity.

2 □ A film such as the following could be shown:
- **a.** A Question of Immunity (16-mm, color, sound, 13-minute film; HAF Alternatives on Film, P.O. Box 22141, San Francisco, CA 94122)
- **b.** Autoimmunity and Disease (16-mm, color, sound, 33-minute film; Merck Sharp and Dohme, Health Information Services Library, West Point, PA 19486)

Evaluation Examples (Test Items)

ESSAY QUESTIONS

1. Discuss points to be considered when evaluating a client for immunization.

2. Outline an active immunization schedule that is usually followed for infants and children in the United States.

3. Describe the normal host-defense system reaction to invading antigens.

UNIT TWELVE: NUTRITIONAL SUPPLEMENTS

43 Oral Supplements

Chapter 43 presents material about a variety of therapeutic agents used to maintain nutritional status: minerals and vitamins, liquid feeding formulas, hematinics, and health food products.

Through the study of this chapter, students may develop the following concepts:

1 □ Nutritional assessment is an important component of nursing care for all clients.
2 □ When the physiologic need for a substance follows a normal distribution, maintenance needs of most people are similar, but there are also people who need much greater or much smaller quantities.
3 □ Deficiencies in nutrients are most frequently multiple rather than single; the most frequent single imbalances are calcium deficiency, iron deficiency, excessive sodium intake, hypervitaminosis A; calcium and iron deficiencies are more likely to develop in women than in men.
4 □ Some nutrients exert pharmacologic effects when administered in large doses.
5 □ A varied balanced diet is the best source of nutrients for most people.
6 □ Minimal daily requirements represent the amount of nutrient needed daily by most people to prevent the development of frank deficiencies.
7 □ Recommended daily allowances are somewhat higher than minimal daily requirements.
8 □ Optimal levels have not been established for intake of many nutrients.
9 □ Supplementation of diet with minerals or vitamins is helpful to persons who have an abnormally high need for them, such as those who absorb nutrients poorly and those who do not consistently eat a varied balanced diet.
10 □ Excessive intake of any nutrient can cause toxicity; safety margins for minerals and fat-soluble vitamins are narrower than those for water-soluble vitamins.
11 □ Birth defects in children are associated with excessive, as well as deficient, nutrient intake.
12 □ Minerals may enter food from the metal of cooking pots.
13 □ Iron deficiency anemia, a hypochromic microcytic anemia, can be caused by inadequate dietary intake of iron, by some condition that results in an increased iron requirement, or by interference with absorption.
14 □ Because of the prevalency of iron deficiency, many foods are iron-fortified, and iron supplements are widely advertised.
15 □ The earliest sign of vitamin B_{12} deficiency is a megaloblastic anemia, but multisystem involvement from this deficiency results in pernicious anemia, which can be fatal if not treated.
16 □ Folic acid deficiency causes a megaloblastic anemia and results from many situations, including the use of certain medications.
17 □ The potency of oral nutritional supplements varies greatly.
18 □ Repeated use of liquid feeding formulas results in taste fatigue and reduced intake; chilling them and offering a variety of preparations delays taste fatigue.
19 □ To prevent dehydration, adequate water must be given to persons receiving concentrated nutritional supplements.

Teaching Strategies

The material in this chapter may be considered in connection with a unit on nutritional needs or with one considering gastrointestinal diseases. Various sections could also be used independently—for example, the section on hematinics could profitably be incorporated into a unit dealing with hypoxia when anemia is covered.

1 □ The class may divide into small groups, with each group developing a table that lists the signs and symptoms of deficiency and toxicity of vitamins and minerals.
2 □ Students may plan and carry out a debate on the following resolution: the use of vitamin and mineral supplements should be limited to people who have abnormally high needs for them, or who cannot absorb them adequately from dietary food.
3 □ As an exercise, students may compute the amount of additional water that should be administered by nasogastric tube to a 200-pound client receiving 250 ml of Isocal qid and oral medications once a day. Project a schedule showing times for feeding, medication, and administering additional water. Be sure students allow for the fluid that is administered

with the feedings and medications for the purpose of flushing the tubing. Consideration should also be given to administering most of the water earlier than late evening to prevent the need to void during the sleeping hours. An example of a suitable schedule that provides a total of 2000 ml of fluid intake would be the following:

7 AM	Formula (250 ml) and water (60 ml)	310 ml
9 AM	Water given with medication	260
11 AM	Water	100
12 noon	Formula and water	310
3 PM	Water	250
5 PM	Formula and water	310
8 PM	Water	150
10 PM	Formula and water	310
		Total 2000 ml

4 □ Have students compare data on mineral or vitamin preparations gathered while completing learning experiences in the drugstore. Analyze the data, considering such questions as the following:

a. How does cost of vitamins and minerals compare with the cost of food sources containing similar doses?

b. Are the doses contained in commercial preparations high enough to encourage toxic intake of nutrients?

c. Should legal restrictions be imposed on the sale of certain over-the-counter preparations?

5 □ Poll your students to determine how many take vitamin and mineral supplements, and the dosages they consume daily. Estimate overall nutrient intake by adding estimated dietary intake. Discuss the implications relative to adequacy of nutrient intake and potential for toxicity.

6 □ Examine the formularies of local health-care agencies to determine the vitamin and mineral preparations adopted for administration to inpatients. Does the written policy specify the vitamin prescriptions for which each should be substituted? What measures are taken to ensure that physicians on the hospital or nursing home staff are aware of these substitutions?

7 □ The following may be considered for discussion:

a. Should everyone eat organ meats rich in vitamins and minerals? How often? If they did, who would eat the leftover portions of the carcasses—steaks, roasts, and so forth?

b. How does the recommended daily allowance for vitamin C intake compare with the recommendations of Linus Pauling? What evidence supports each viewpoint? Discuss possible risks associated with following each recommendation.

c. Can vegetarian diets provide adequate mineral and vitamin nutrition without risk of toxicity? Consider strict vegetarian regimens as well as lacto-ovovegetarian regimens.

d. Discuss human requirements for iron, vitamin B_{12}, and folic acid. What types of situations can increase the body's need for each of these hematinics? Identify specific foods that can provide each of the three substances.

e. Discuss the types of anemias that can occur with deficiencies of each of the above hematinics. Describe the diagnostic tools and the treatment regimens used. Explain what points would be outlined for clients and these problems in your teaching plans for them.

8 □ Compare costs of nationally advertised brands of vitamin and mineral supplements with "house" brands offered for sale, using data that students have gathered in the drug store.

9 □ Open a vitamin capsule and encourage students to smell and taste the contents. Discuss ingredients used in the preparation of supplements, such as fish liver oils and brewers' yeast.

10 □ If there are known vegetarians in the local population, invite one or more to address the class to explain their dietary beliefs and practices. If skin tones reflect high carotene levels, discuss this effect of vegetarian regimens.

Evaluation Examples (Test Items)

SHORT ANSWER QUESTIONS

1. Define the following nutritional terms:

Vitamin	Scurvy
Mineral	Minimal daily requirement
Electrolyte	Recommended daily allowance
Xerophthalmia	
Pellagra	

2. Identify the two vitamins most likely to produce toxicity when administered in doses greater than the recommended daily allowance.

MULTIPLE CHOICE ITEMS

1. High levels of carotene in the diet produce
- a. An orange yellow coloration of the skin
- b. A deficiency of vitamin A
- c. A degree of protection against the development of xerophthalmia

1. a, b
*2. a, c
3. b, c
4. All of the above

2. Nutritional deficiencies are most likely to develop in clients with
*1. Sprue
2. Constipation
3. Recent cessation of smoking
4. Hypothyroidism

3. Alcoholics have an increased need for
1. Sugar
2. Vitamin A
*3. Vitamin B complex
4. Vitamin K

4. Two minerals currently employed medically for drug effect are

a. Arsenic
b. Calcium
c. Lithium

1. a, b
2. a, c
*3. b, c
4. All of the above

5. The most prevalent mineral deficiency in the United States is deficiency of

1. Calcium
2. Zinc
3. Copper
4. Sodium
*5. Iron

6. A typical pathophysiologic reason for pernicious anemia is

1. Dietary deficiency of vitamin B_{12}
*2. Failure of parietal cell function
3. Neurologic dysfunction
4. Atypical erythrocyte production

7. One reason parenteral iron would be selected for use is that

1. Response to parenteral iron is faster than response to oral iron
*2. Iron stores may be more rapidly created with parenteral iron than with oral iron
3. Compliance with parenteral iron therapy is better than with oral therapy
4. Intolerance of oral iron preparations is very high

8. The usual dose of iron sulfate administered for iron deficiency is about

1. 300 μg
2. 3 mg
*3. 300 mg
4. 3 g

9. Z-track technique should be used when administering injections of

1. Fat-soluble vitamins
2. Water-soluble vitamins
3. Vitamin B_{12}
*4. Iron

10. Folic-acid deficiency can occur because the diet is deficient in this substance. The diet may be deficient because

1. The client is trying to lose weight and is avoiding foods high in calories
*2. Protracted cooking can destroy 90% of a food's folate content
3. The client dislikes milk and most milk products
4. The foods high in folate content tend to be the more expensive ones on a shopping list

11. To prevent harmful side effects from use of potassium supplements, these preparations should be administered

1. Between meals, on an empty stomach
2. Parenterally, by intramuscular or intravenous injection
3. Intravenously, by slow infusion
*4. With ample amounts of fluid

12. The Schilling test is used to diagnose a disease characterized by deficiency of

1. Iron
2. Copper
3. Vitamin A
*4. Vitamin B_{12}

44 Parenteral Preparations

Parenteral Fluids
Clear Solutions
Nursing Management
Nursing Implications
Nursing Process
Total Parenteral Nutrition
Nursing Management
Nursing Implications
Nursing Process
Blood
Nursing Management
Nursing Implications
Nursing Process

Chapter 44 discusses parenteral fluids and blood transfusions.

Through the study of this chapter, students may develop the following concepts:

1 □ To prevent tissue damage, both hypotonic and hypertonic parenteral fluids must be administered slowly and infused into as large a vein as possible.

2 □ Parenteral administration of nutritional supplements poses risks of serious infection and physiologic imbalance; the administration of blood involves additional risks of clotting disorders and antigen–antibody reactions.

3 □ Before administration, blood must be typed and cross-matched for ABO and Rh compatibility; special precautions must be taken to prevent the administration of mismatched blood.

4 □ Some degree of antigen–antibody reaction occurs whenever transfused blood is not identical in type to that of the recipient; the most serious reactions occur when the recipient's serum contains antibodies against transfused erythrocytes.

5 □ Autotransfusions are safer than homologous transfusions; whenever possible, clients should donate their own blood in preparation for elective procedures during which blood is likely to be needed.

Teaching Strategies

The material in this chapter is appropriate for consideration in connection with a unit on nutritional needs, parenteral therapy, or life-threatening illness.

1 □ If there is a recipient of parenteral nutrition in the community who is not disabled (such as a young, otherwise healthy person with Crohn's disease), invite him or her to visit a class and share with students the impact of this therapy on lifestyle.

2 □ The policies and procedures for administering blood that have been established by one or more acute care facilities may be evaluated, comparing these policies with one another or with guidelines from textbooks, assessing their strengths and weaknesses. If local practices have deficiencies, develop model policies and procedures suitable for use in local agencies.

3 □ The following may be considered for discussion:

a. What qualities and characteristics would be required of an artificial substitute for blood?

b. Compare the advantages and disadvantages of blood as a therapeutic agent.

4 □ Divide the class into two groups. Have these groups prepare to debate the pros and cons of the following: *Resolved:* The practice of buying blood for blood banks should be banned in favor of complete reliance on donated blood.

Evaluation Examples (Test Items)

SITUATION-BASED MULTIPLE CHOICE ITEMS

Situation: You are caring for Mr. WA, a debilitated client hospitalized for surgery to relieve obstruction of the esophagus caused by cancer. To improve his nutritional status, he is receiving a hyperalimentation solution in a central venous line and Intralipid infusion in a peripheral vein.

1. The hyperalimentation solution is infused into the vena cava because it is
1. Hypotonic
*2. Hypertonic
3. Isotonic
4. Extremely irritating to the veins

2. The therapeutic response expected from administration of the nutritional infusions is
1. Prevention of further weight loss
2. Correction of metabolic alkalosis
3. Correction of water intoxication
*4. An increase in body mass

3. An adverse reaction likely to develop in WA is (are)
1. Thromboemboli
*2. Infection with septicemia
3. Metabolic acidosis
4. Hypoglycemia

4. WA should be assessed regularly for
a. Glycosuria
b. Septicemia
c. Changes in body weight
1. a, b
2. a, c
3. b, c
*4. All of the above

5. Before administering Intralipid, the nurse should
1. Agitate the container to ensure even distribution of the fat
2. Warm the solution to body temperature
*3. Inspect the solution for separation
4. Add a surfactant compound to the solution to ensure homogeneity

Situation: You are caring for Ms. CM, a 50-year-old secretary who has a history of dysfunctional bleeding for 2 years. She has experienced protracted, heavy menstrual flow for 4 weeks that did not respond to hormonal therapy. A hysterectomy has been scheduled, and she is to receive 2 units of packed red blood cells to replace lost blood.

1. Before hanging the blood, the nurse should verify that the unit of packed cells delivered to the nursing ward has been properly typed and cross-matched for CM by
1. Checking the physician's order for blood
2. Comparing the label on the unit of RBCs with CM's identification armband
3. Requesting that a technician from the blood laboratory check the identity of the unit of RBCs in his or her presence
*4. Requesting that another nurse check the identity of the unit of RBCs in his or her presence

2. After starting infusion of the blood, the nurse should
1. Instruct the client to call a nurse immediately if she experiences any discomfort
*2. Keep the client under direct observation until 50 ml of blood has infused
3. Keep the client under direct observation until all of the blood has infused
4. Verify that adrenalin is available at the bedside for use in case of a transfusion reaction

3. How much time must elapse after a transfusion before the client may be reassured that she will have no adverse reaction to the transfusion?
1. No time; after completion of the transfusion with no adverse effect, the client may be reassured
2. 48 hours
3. 6 months, if her blood tests negative for hepatitis B antibodies
*4. 2 years, if her blood tests negative for HIV antibodies

4. If CM refuses the transfusion, what is the nurse's best response?
1. Tell CM that the transfusion is necessary for safe completion of her surgery
2. Tell CM that the surgery may be postponed until her blood has been replaced by natural processes
*3. Tell CM that new techniques might be used to prevent another menstrual cycle and to stimulate red blood cell replacement
4. Agree with CM that transfusions are dangerous treatments

UNIT THIRTEEN: MISCELLANEOUS DRUG FAMILIES

45
Diagnostic Agents

Radiopaque Contrast Media
Barium Sulfate
Iodinated Contrast Media
Nursing Management
Agents Used for Volumetric Diagnostic Tests
Nonradioactive Compounds
Radioactive Tracers
Provocative Agents
Nursing Management
Dermal Reactivity Indicators
Nursing Management

For purposes of discussion, Chapter 45 classifies diagnostic agents into the following categories: radiopaque media, polysaccharides and dyes used for volumetric testing, radioactive tracers, provocative agents, and dermal reactivity indicators. This division allows discussion of properties and client responses common to drugs within each group.

Through the study of this chapter, students may develop the following concepts:

1 □ Substances administered for diagnostic purposes pose risks of adverse reaction by clients.
2 □ All exposure to ionizing radiation is cumulative over a person's lifetime; no level of exposure can be considered "safe."
3 □ Tracer doses of radionuclides involve minimal exposure to ionizing radiation compared with the more dangerous high-level exposure of therapeutic doses of radionuclides.
4 □ The risks of toxicity caused by ionizing radiation of tracer doses are much greater for persons repeatedly exposed to such doses in the course of their occupations than for clients receiving them occasionally for diagnostic purposes.
5 □ Drugs administered for local effect in the gastrointestinal tract can cause adverse reactions, even when they are relatively unreactive in the tract.
6 □ Care must be taken to differentiate between medicinally useful and poisonous substances that have similar names (*e.g.*, barium sulfate and barium sulfite).
7 □ Provocative diagnostic agents can cause serious adverse reactions, especially when clients have a disease whose signs and symptoms are elicited or exaggerated during the test.
8 □ Accuracy in carrying out diagnostic tests is critical for the generation of reliable data.
9 □ Clients undergoing diagnostic tests experience high levels of stress because of apprehension about their diagnoses.
10 □ Dermal skin reactivity tests to diagnose allergy are conducted only when skilled medical personnel are available to treat serious adverse reactions.

Teaching Strategies

1 □ Students involved with clinical practice should accompany clients and observe diagnostic studies in progress. Their impressions of and reactions to these tests may be discussed in clinical postconference or in class.
2 □ Obtain a supply of a barium sulfate preparation used for oral doses during radiography. Allow students to examine the liquid. If any students have experience with radiography involving barium administration, have them describe their impressions of and reactions to the test.
3 □ Arrange a tour of a center for nuclear medicine, guided by a person knowledgeable about nuclear safety.

SITUATION-BASED MULTIPLE CHOICE ITEMS

Situation: Mr. SC, a 52-year-old accountant, has had intermittent diarrhea for several weeks. He is scheduled to have a barium enema done as an outpatient procedure tomorrow morning. Standard preparation for this procedure involves administration of a laxative (castor oil) the afternoon before the test, and enemas until clear the morning of the test.

1. Before instructing SC about preparation for the test, you should determine
1. Whether he is currently having diarrheal stools
2. Whether SC knows how to administer an enema
*3. Both of the above

2. SC tells you that he is having five or six watery stools a day, and that he feels weak. You should
1. Tell SC to omit the laxative ordered as part of the preparation
2. Tell SC to omit the enemas before the test
3. Caution SC to omit neither the laxative nor the enemas
*4. Ask the physician whether the laxative should be given

3. SC wonders what the x-ray examination will be like. You should tell him that he will be given
1. A thick drink somewhat like a milk shake that has a chalky taste
2. An intravenous injection that may cause him to feel warm and flushed
*3. An enema that will later be drained from the colon
4. A brassy-tasting solution to drink

4. You should warn SC that, after the test,

*1. Some barium may appear as gray streaks in the stools
2. He may break out in a slight skin rash
3. The barium may make his diarrhea temporarily worse
4. All of the above

5. To prevent an adverse reaction to the barium, you would advise SC to

1. Take soft, easily digested food low in fiber
2. Fast for several hours after the test
3. Watch for tarry stools
*4. Drink plenty of water and use a laxative if he becomes at all constipated

Situation: Ms. BG, age 40 years, is scheduled to have a gallbladder series in the hospital next week.

1. Before giving BG the iodinated contrast dye she will be taking the night before the test, you should ask her

1. Whether she has ever had similar procedures using radiopaque dyes
2. Whether she has ever had an adverse reaction to iodine or radiopaque dyes
3. How often she has been exposed to x-rays or other radiation in the past
*4. All of the above

2. In relation to the radiopaque dye,

a. She should take an enema the day before the test
b. It is important to take all the medication
c. The instructions regarding the timing of the medication should be followed exactly

1. a, b
2. a, c
*3. b, c
4. All of the above

3. The afternoon after the test has been performed, BG calls you to report that she has broken out in a fine red "itchy" rash. You should tell her that

1. The rash is probably unrelated to the test
2. This is a common occurrence following a test using iodine-containing radiopaque dyes, and is of no consequence
*3. She should consider herself allergic to iodine and radiopaque dyes, and should carry a medical identification device warning of this
4. She should go immediately to an emergency medical facility because an anaphylactic reaction could occur

Situation: LS, a 6-year-old girl, is to be skin-tested for allergy to determine what substances she is sensitive to. Her mother wants to know what the tests will be like (the physician uses scratch tests).

1. You would tell her mother that

1. LS will be given a series of intradermal injections with a short needle
2. A series of scratches will be made on LS's skin, and patches similar to Band-Aids will be applied for a short time
3. LS's skin will be pressed firmly with a device that has several tines to produce minute scratches in the skin
*4. LS's skin will be scratched with a small instrument, after which a solution will be applied to the site

2. Her mother wishes to know how long the tests will take. You should tell her that the office visit will

1. Probably be short, because the tests take only a few minutes
*2. Be quite long, because a number of tests are usually required, and the results cannot be determined immediately
3. Be somewhat longer than usual, but the test results will not be determined until a later visit

3. Her mother asks if the tests will hurt. You should tell her that

a. The scratching is uncomfortable but not painful
b. Itching and redness will probably occur at some of the sites
c. There is a small chance of a mild systemic allergic reaction, but that this rarely happens because of the small dosage used
d. There is no risk of a serious allergic reaction

*1. a, b, c
2. a, b, d
3. a, c, d
4. b, c, d
5. All of the above

46
Enzymes and Drugs Affecting Enzymes

Chapter 46 discusses enzymes, enzyme inhibitors, and enzyme reactivators. The role played by these drugs in current medical practice, the risk of allergic reactions, and the prospects of future uses in the correction of genetic defects in metabolism are indicated. In addition, data on drugs of this type not discussed in other chapters of the book are given.

This chapter will probably be most useful to students as a reference; however, it could be used to illustrate the following concepts:

1 □ Drugs acting as enzymes (particularly those derived from nonhuman sources) tend to produce allergic sensitivity and often cause anaphylaxis on repeated exposure.
2 □ Drugs must be delivered to the site of action before they can produce a therapeutic effect.
3 □ Allergy to drugs is an occupational hazard for nurses; nurses should avoid contact with drugs such as enzymes that are antigenic.

Teaching Strategies

This chapter will be used by most instructors only as a source for drug data; however, class discussion could consider such questions as the following:

1 □ What are the signs and symptoms of anaphylaxis? How is this condition treated?
2 □ How can the nurse best gather a history of allergy to drugs?
3 □ What procedures are used to gain permission for treatment when the client cannot give consent and treatment cannot be delayed?

Evaluation Examples (Test Items)

ESSAY QUESTIONS

1. Outline the points to be covered in a teaching plan to educate a client about disulfiram therapy.

2. Briefly discuss the appropriate nursing actions to take once a client is identified as lactose intolerant.

MULTIPLE CHOICE ITEMS

1. Common adverse reactions to the use of chymopapain include
- a. Prolonged muscle stiffness
- b. Allergic sensitivity to papaya
- c. Altered touch sensations
- d. Anaphylaxis
- *1. a, b, c
- 2. a, b, d
- 3. a, c, d
- 4. b, c, d

2. Clients who are to receive pralidoxime should be screened for
- 1. Unhealed bone fractures
- 2. Orthostatic hypotension
- 3. Calcified gallstones
- *4. Myasthenia gravis

3. Clients who are on a drug regimen of disulfiram must avoid ingesting
- 1. Hard cheeses
- *2. Alcohol
- 3. Chianti wine
- 4. Wine vinegar

4. Lactase is usually administered
- 1. Orally
- 2. By injection
- 3. Topically
- *4. It is not administered to the client directly but is added to milk prior to consumption

47
Complexes: Chelators and Ion-Exchange Compounds

Chelators
Ion-Exchange Compounds

Chapter 47 discusses medications that act by exchanging ions with, or chelating chemicals that are potentially harmful to, the body so that the harmful elements are eliminated from the body. Some of these drugs (antacids and hypocholesteremics) are discussed in detail in other chapters. This chapter will probably be most useful as reference material; however, it could be used to illustrate the following concepts:

1 □ Drugs acting locally in the gastrointestinal tract may affect nutrition and cause serious systemic adverse reactions (*e.g.*, trace mineral deficiency that can cause birth defects in exposed fetuses).
2 □ Manipulation of the internal chemical environment, which may be helpful in the treatment of disease conditions, may also cause serious adverse reactions.

Teaching Strategies

This chapter will be used by most instructors only as a source for drug data. It could, however, be studied in a unit on toxicology in relation to the treatment of heavy metal poisoning.

Evaluation Examples (Test Items)

MULTIPLE CHOICE ITEMS

1. A metal that is *not* removed from the body by dimercaprol is
  a. Arsenic
  *b. Calcium
  c. Gold
  d. Lead

2. A drug used to lower serum potassium levels in renal failure is
  a. Cholestyramine
  b. Aluminum hydroxide
  *c. Sodium polystyrene sulfonate
  d. Penicillamine

3. A drug used in the treatment of lead poisoning is
  *a. Edetate calcium disodium
  b. Edetate disodium
  c. Deferoxamine mesylate
  d. Cholestyramine

UNIT FOURTEEN: SPECIAL CONSIDERATIONS IN DRUG THERAPY

48
Substance Abuse

Nature of Dependence and Addiction
Definition of Terms
Circles of Dependence
Classifications
Commonly Abused Substances
Opioid Analgesics
General Central Nervous System Depressants
Alcohol
Central Nervous System Sympathomimetics (Adrenergics)
Nicotine
Cannabinoids
Psychedelics
Other Substances of Abuse
Substance Control
Nursing Management
Nursing Implications
Nursing Process

Chapter 48 introduces the student to the problems of abuse of pharmacologically active substances. The text describes the major categories of drug abuse and discusses in detail the pharmacologic effects of each drug classification, the potential for the development of tolerance or dependence, and treatment modalities used in current detoxification and rehabilitation programs. The student is exposed to various concepts related to the psychosocial and physiologic ramifications of substance use and abuse. In addition, a framework for the classification of addiction is discussed.

A study of the material presented will allow the student to develop the following concepts:

1 □ The professional nurse appreciates the nature and scope of substance abuse and develops a sensitivity to the physical, emotional, psychologic, developmental, and social consequences of drug-related dependency.

2 □ There are seven major groups of commonly abused substances. Each can be differentiated in relationship to general pharmacologic effects by the nature of tolerance or by dependence in each category.

3 □ Each category has therapeutic interventions that have been proven to be most useful in treatment of drug intoxication or withdrawal in that category.

4 □ The professional nurse understands the mechanisms set forth by the federal government for control of specific substances.

Teaching Strategies

Given the current statistics regarding the prevalence of substance abuse in the American population, it is realistic to expect that many students will have had varying degrees of experience with substance abuse, whether legal or illicit. Inviting exploration of personal life habits may provide an opportunity to discuss the attitudes, feelings, and values that accompany decision making in relation to personal choices. Discussing habitual behavior common to activities of daily living and the efforts required to alter these habits may establish greater sensitivity to the impact of substance abuse on one's life.

1 □ Chapter 49, pertaining to drugs (nicotine and alcohol) used during pregnancy and lactation, may be used as reference material or may become part of the discussion class.

2 □ Local drug enforcement agencies maintain several teaching aids, including films and exhibits of illicit substances and drug paraphernalia. Speakers are usually available to facilitate discussion following a group presentation.

3 □ Presentation of a panel discussion to include drug counselors, crisis center workers, former addicts, and alcoholics provides students with the opportunity to obtain firsthand knowledge from the victims of abuse.

4 □ Assignment of the Learning Experiences will provide basic information for students to use in class discussion. The availability of community-based observations may require selective assignment of the learning activities.

Evaluation Examples (Test Items)

SHORT ANSWER ESSAY QUESTIONS

1. Define and differentiate the following terms:

Abuse	Drug dependence
Addiction	Drug tolerance

2. Describe the four phases of the opiate withdrawal syndrome.

3. Identify and describe the four circles of drug dependence and addiction.

4. Describe the three stages of the alcohol withdrawal syndrome.

MULTIPLE CHOICE ITEMS

1. The state that exists when a client feels the compulsion to maintain continuous use of a substance for the desired effect is called
1. Abuse
*2. Psychologic dependence
3. Tolerance
4. Addiction

2. Which of the following is true about the nature of drug dependence?
1. Addictive behavior is dependent on the original motivating force
2. During the initial period of drug abuse, the user cannot control consumption
*3. The more potent a chemical agent, the more rapidly addiction develops
4. A negative relationship exists between potency and dependency

3. According to Bejerot's classification of addiction, therapeutic addiction
a. May be a consequence of medical treatment
b. Is frequently contagious
c. Is the most common type in the Western world
d. Most commonly occurs among health personnel
1. a only
*2. a, d
3. b, d
4. c only

4. The pharmacologic effects of opioid analgesics include
a. Pinpoint pupils, decreased vision, short-lived euphoria
b. Sleep, nausea, vomiting, respiratory depression with large doses
c. Warm flushed skin
d. Poor memory, impaired thinking, slurred speech
*1. a, b, c
2. b, d
3. a, c
4. All of the above

5. Which of the following is *not* true regarding central nervous system depressants?
*1. Tolerance occurs slowly
2. Withdrawal syndrome is more severe than a narcotic withdrawal syndrome
3. Symptoms of abstinence are evident within 24 hours after the drug is discontinued
4. Physical and psychologic dependence results from excessive and prolonged use

6. In the metabolism of alcohol, which of the following is *not* true?
1. Occurs at a rate of 10 ml per hour in an average adult
2. Affects the secretory and motor functions of the gastrointestinal tract
*3. Acts as a central nervous system stimulant
4. Produces constipation or diarrhea with immoderate use

7. Legal evidence of alcohol intoxication in most states is
*1. 0.10% blood alcohol level
2. 0.05% blood alcohol level
3. 0.50% blood alcohol level
4. 0.25% blood alcohol level

8. Chronic toxic doses of amphetamines may lead to which of the following symptoms?
a. Compulsive, repetitive body movements
b. Facial grimacing
c. Passive withdrawal
d. Death resulting from extremes of heat or exercise
1. a, b
2. a, c
*3. a, b, d
4. All of the above

9. The estimated ranking of the most commonly abused substances in the United States today is (from most abused to least)
1. Caffeine, nicotine, alcohol, marijuana
2. Alcohol, caffeine, marijuana, nicotine
*3. Nicotine, alcohol, caffeine, marijuana
4. Caffeine, nicotine, marijuana, alcohol

MATCHING QUESTION

1. Phencyclidine (PCP)	A or C	A. DOA
2. Amphetamine	D	B. Smack
3. Methaqualone	F	C. Angel dust
4. Heroin	B	D. Black beauty
5. Cocaine	E	E. Nose candy
		F. Soaper

49 Drug Therapy in Maternal Care

Drug Use in Pregnancy
Nonmedical Factors Affecting Pregnancy Medications
Nursing Management
Nursing Implications
Nursing Process
Drug Use During Labor
Premature Labor
Induction of Labor
Pain Control During Labor
Drug Use During Delivery
Other Drugs Used During Labor
Local/Regional Anesthetics
General Anesthetics
Drug Use During Postpartum Care
Nursing Management
Nursing Implications
Drug Use During Lactation
Breast-Feeding
Maternal Medications and the Lactating Woman
Nursing Management
Nursing Implications
Nursing Process

Chapter 49 is divided into five main phases of maternal health care: pregnancy, labor, delivery, postpartum period, and lactation. The use of drugs in these phases and how they affect both mother and fetus are examined, along with nursing management in the care of mother and fetus (infant).

Maternal nutrition during pregnancy affects the mother's well-being, the growth and development of the fetus, and the preparation of the mother's breasts for lactation. She needs education about the quantity and quality of her diet, and information about the dangers of drugs (including alcohol and over-the-counter preparations) that she may be using.

The fetus is an unwitting recipient of material that travels to it from the maternal circulatory system through the placenta. The fetal concentration of substances may reach 50% to 100% of those in the mother, possibly higher if detoxification is inadequate, or if the substances are excreted into the amniotic fluid and then ingested and recirculated in the fetus. The chapter documents the fetal tissues that are particularly receptive to specific drugs, as well as drugs with known or suspected teratogenic, mutagenic, carcinogenic, or other effects. Cigarette smoke has been implicated in higher incidences of placental problems (abruptio and previa), as well as in low birth weights, retardation, and slow growth.

On the other hand, drugs may be needed to treat a maternal medical disorder. Because most drugs can be transferred to the fetus through the placenta, evaluation of the possible effects of maternal disorders and maternal medication on the fetus is imperative. There is also information on the administration of drugs to the mother as a method of intervention in fetal medical problems.

The pregnancy section of the chapter should be thoroughly reviewed by students who are caring for antepartum clients.

The second section of the chapter traces the changes in management of those clients in premature labor from the period prior to the 1970s, when care did not change the course of neonatal respiratory disease syndrome, to the 1980s. Currently, the administration of tocolytic agents and corticosteroids to pregnant women has proven highly successful as a way of inducing fetal pulmonary maturation. The chapter also presents material to demonstrate possible conflicts between maternal and fetal interests. For example, the use of oxytocic drugs may be helpful to the laboring mother, but may cause cardiac arrhythmias or cerebral damage in the neonate. Drugs used for maternal analgesia or sedation may lead to neonatal respiratory depression. Epidural anesthesia may do away with the pain of labor, but may result in a forceps or cesarean delivery. Even pain control following delivery has to be evaluated for its effects on the nursing neonate.

Students assigned to labor and delivery units would benefit from a review of this section.

The final portion of the chapter explores some issues involved in the maternal decision to breast- or formula-feed the newborn, and also presents information on the possibility of deleterious effects of many commonly used drugs on the infant. This information in and of itself is insufficient because new drugs are introduced frequently. Therefore, information on how to evaluate the possible effects of any drug on the infant is presented. This includes the method of administration to the mother, the way in which the drug is transported to the child, the effect of a drug's molecular weight, ionization, and solubility, the storage of the substance in the baby's system, and the ability of the infant to detoxify and excrete the drug from its body.

It would be helpful to students who are studying obstetric nursing to study this chapter. At the same time, the instructor should remember that such students are often young, and females may identify closely with the new mothers for whom they are caring. Many, if not most, first-time mothers are in a very vulnerable position in terms of motherhood, particularly when breast-feeding. They often are not prepared for the fact that breast-feeding is a learned art and skill, not "second nature." These new mothers should be thoroughly supported in their efforts to breast-feed. Of course, they should be advised appropriately about precautions to take when medications must be taken. However, students should be cautioned about the negative impact that too many discouraging statements or warnings can have on the neophyte mother who wants the best for her baby and who is easily alarmed. Instructors assigning this chapter should emphasize the student care-giver's importance to the new mother.

Through the study of this chapter, the student may develop the following concepts:

1 □ Proper nutrition is important to both the pregnant woman and the fetus during pregnancy for maternal health, healthy fetal development, and preparation for breast-feeding.

2 □ Maternal medications may be valuable or dangerous to the fetus.

3 □ Maternal drugs may be teratogenic, mutagenic, or carcinogenic to the fetus.

4 □ Both cigarettes and alcohol may be harmful to the fetus.

5 □ There is a possible conflict of health and comfort interests between the mother and her unborn child when administration of medications is considered, and the nurse must recognize the pregnant woman's personal needs while helping her adjust her lifestyle to fetal needs.

6 □ The responsible nurse provides accurate information so that clients can make valid judgments about the use of medications for their comfort during labor and delivery.

7 □ Evaluation of the route of maternal administration and the period of time the drug is to be taken may be made in relation to the effect of the drug on the infant.

8 □ The ability of the infant to detoxify and excrete various substances varies with age or stages of maturity.

9 □ There is a relationship between a drug's molecular weight, ionization, and solubility and its ability to affect the child.

10 □ The professional nurse can learn to determine the effects on the infant of a specific drug administered to a lactating woman.

Teaching Strategies

1 □ Classroom discussion may be stimulated by the following questions:

- **a.** What are the five major considerations that can be used to evaluate possible fetal harm resulting from maternal drug administration?
- **b.** The pregnant nurse is exposed to medical substances that may be harmful to her fetus. Discuss how nurses should protect themselves in the work place.
- **c.** Contrast the medical and nonmedical treatments of nausea and vomiting associated with early pregnancy.
- **d.** Plan a teaching program for a group of pregnant clients who want an evaluation of analgesic drugs commonly used during labor and delivery.
- **e.** Describe four situations for which induction of labor might be considered.
- **f.** Discuss the section of the public health law in New York State that orders physicians and nurse-midwives to "inform the expectant mother, in advance of the birth, of the drugs that such physician (nurse-midwife) expects to employ during pregnancy and . . . at birth, and of the possible effects of such drugs on the child and mother."
- **g.** Name several substances transported from mother to child through the mother's milk that are advantageous to the newborn (vitamins C and K, various amino acids, thyroid for infants with hypothyroidism).
- **h.** Under what conditions should a mother be discouraged from breast-feeding (infant with galactosemia, some maternal illnesses)?
- **i.** Describe three possible reactions of the nursing infant to maternal medications (rash, drowsiness, irritability, diarrhea).

2 □ Students may design posters for placement in an antepartum clinic. Possible subjects include smoking, nutrition, alcohol, recreational drugs, over-the-counter drug use (aspirin, cough medicine), and information about maternal conditions requiring the use of medications.

3 □ Role play may focus on the nurse educating a client or a group of clients on the need to refrain from smoking during pregnancy.

Evaluation Examples (Test Items)

ESSAY QUESTIONS

1. Prepare a plan for educating women on the effects of alcoholism on the fetus. Include information on maternal detoxification.

2. Describe the changes in the liver that affect drug metabolism during pregnancy.

3. Describe how changes in maternal blood and plasma volume during pregnancy affect the transfer of drugs from mother to fetus.

4. Discuss the potential dangers, as well as the benefits, to mother and fetus from the use of ritodrine.

5. Outline an approach that can be used when caring for the following client:

- **a.** A woman who wants a drug-free delivery but must have gas anesthesia for an immediate forceps delivery because of fetal distress.
- **b.** A woman who is refused medication for pain relief because of fetal bradycardia.

6. Discuss the use of RH_0(D) immune globulin in relation to a delivery, including prenatal administration for women at risk.

7. Discuss the way in which atropine sulfate may be taken unwittingly by the pregnant woman (constituent of over-the-counter drugs or prescribed medication), and how it then affects the baby. Include information on molecular weight, ionization, method of transport, metabolism, detoxification, and excretion.

8. Discuss the factors to be considered for the nursing infant when anticoagulants are ordered for the mother. Compare the possible effects of phenindione, ethyl biscoumacetate, and the coumarin derivatives on the baby.

9. Compare the possible effects on a nursing infant of aspirin, acetaminophen, and propoxyphene if they are taken by the newly delivered mother.

MULTIPLE CHOICE ITEMS

1. Which of the following metabolic changes may affect drugs prior to crossing the placenta?
  a. Oxidation
  b. Reduction
  c. Dealkylation
  d. Synthesis
  1. a, d
  2. b, c
  3. c, d
  4. a, c
  *5. All of the above

2. Choose the correct combination of drugs and receptive fetal tissue from the following list:
  a. Vagina—diethylstilbesterol
  b. Otic nerve—streptomycin
  c. Platelets—aspirin
  d. Red blood cells—digoxin
  e. Central nervous system—warfarin
  *1. a, b, c
  2. b, c, d
  3. a, b, e
  4. a, c, d
  5. All of the above

3. Which of the following drugs may be given to the mother to treat fetal conditions?
  a. Sodium levothyroxine
  b. Biotin
  c. Glucocorticoids
  d. Penicillin
  e. Digoxin
  1. a, e
  2. b, c
  3. d, e
  4. c, d
  *5. All of the above

4. Before the 1970s, premature labor was managed with which of the following?
  a. Avoidance of sexual activity
  b. Tocolytic drugs
  c. Sedation
  d. Ethanol
  e. Oxytocic drugs
  1. a, b
  *2. a, c
  3. a, d
  4. a, e
  5. All of the above

5. Which of the following drugs are used in the treatment of convulsions during labor?
  a. Magnesium sulfate
  b. Meperidine hydrochloride
  c. Promethazine hydrochloride
  d. Phenobarbital
  1. b, c
  2. b, d
  3. a, c
  *4. a, d
  5. All of the above

6. Drugs with which of the following characteristics can be expected to pass through breast milk?
  a. Molecular weight over 200
  b. Fat-soluble large molecules
  c. Ionized molecules
  d. Molecular weight under 200
  e. Fat-soluble small molecules
  1. a, b
  2. b, c
  *3. b, d
  4. c, e
  5. d, e

7. Drugs are most likely to be transported into milk passively by
  a. Proteins
  b. Sodium
  c. Carrier enzymes
  d. Glucose
  e. Fat-soluble substances
  1. a, b
  *2. a, c
  3. b, d
  4. c, e
  5. d, e

8. Which of the following antibiotics given to the mothers have little, if any, effect on the nursing infant?
  a. Erythromycin
  b. Cephalothin
  c. Oxacillin
  d. Sulfanilamide
  e. Lincomycin
  1. c, d, e
  2. a, c, e
  3. b, c, d
  *4. b, c, e
  5. All of the above

50
Drug Therapy in Pediatric Nursing

Determining the Appropriate Dosage
Factors Influencing Response
Uniqueness of the Individual
Body System Maturity and Metabolism
Pharmacologic Toxicity
Genetic Endowment
Chronic Conditions
Circadian Rhythms
Psychological Development
Factors in Administering Medications
Infants
Toddlers
Preschoolers
School-Aged Children
Adolescents
Nursing Management
Nursing Implications
Nursing Process

Chapter 50 considers the pediatric client as a unique individual with many special considerations when medications are administered. Appropriate dosages are determined by the use of rules, ratios, and formulas to facilitate safe medication administration. The influence on the child's health state and reaction to pharmaceutic agents of age, genetic endowment, body system maturity and metabolism, level of wellness, and environment are considered. Psychological development influences the nurse's approach to medication administration and the child's knowledge and acceptance of a therapeutic regimen. Using a foundation of developmental theory, approaches to medication administration are explored. The use of play and play therapy as helpful nursing interventions are discussed in the chapter. The professional nurse and the pediatric patient benefit from a blend of knowledge in the art of administering medications to infants and young children and the scientific base of physiology, pathophysiology, developmental theories, and pharmacology.

Through the study of the chapter, the student may develop the following concepts:

1 □ The administration of medications to infants and children requires knowledge of their unique physical and psychological development.
2 □ Appropriate dosages are determined by the use of published and professional resources and predetermined formulas.
3 □ Infants and children respond in unique ways to medication based on body system maturity, age, genetic endowment, health state, psychological development, and environment.
4 □ The renal system of young infants contains fewer glomeruli and lacks efficient excretion of certain substances. The risk of cumulative toxicity is increased in this age group.
5 □ Cumulative effects of medication may be enhanced in the presence of chronic illness, dehydration, depleted nutritional state, and via inherited factors.
6 □ Chronic illness may affect a child's psychological well-being and acceptance of prolonged use of medications.
7 □ The chronically ill child may require multiple drug therapy with increased risk of adverse drug reactions.
8 □ Knowledge of developmental theory and its practical applications to the pediatric client will assist the nurse in medication administration.
9 □ A therapeutic relationship between the child, parent, and nurse will facilitate pharmaceutic interventions.
10 □ Play functions as an explorative medium that aids the child in understanding and integrating therapeutic interventions.
11 □ Advocating for the pediatric client is within the role of the professional nurse.
12 □ The professional nurse uses the nursing process to collect a data base with the goal of assessing, planning, and implementing an individualized plan of care for the pediatric client and family; evaluation is a continual process and may include input from the nurse, child, and family.

Teaching Strategies

1 □ Assign the students to groups of three to five members. Each group should choose one of the following: infants, toddlers, preschoolers, school-age children, and young adolescents. The students are to determine safe and effective methods of administering oral and intramuscular medications to the well, acutely ill, and chronically ill child. Factors such as growth and development, maturity of organ systems, height, weight and body surface data, experience with the health-care system, type, form, and palatability of medication, and average prescribed dosages should be considered. Discussion of these methods can follow lecture–classroom discussions or preclinical conferences prior to experiences on pediatric units, well-child clinics, or ambulatory outpatient settings. Role playing may also be helpful.
2 □ While caring for a sick child during the pediatric experience, the student will formulate a care plan focusing on teaching the child and parents about the child's medications. Previously used over-the-counter and currently prescribed medications will be included in the plan. Encourage the child and parents to ask questions about medications. Discuss safety measures for medications when the child returns home. Care plans may be shared within the clinical group to foster discussion on methods to administer medications to

different age children. Determine whether the prescribed doses of medications are appropriate to the individual child and his level of development. Discuss the legal and professional implications for the professional nurse if children are receiving pharmaceutical products inappropriate for their body weight or organ maturation.

Through role playing, explore approaches to discuss incorrect doses with other health-care providers.

Evaluation Examples (Test Items)

ESSAY QUESTIONS

1. Identify six factors that may influence an infant's or child's response to a given medication. Describe how four of these factors affect pharmaceutic products in the pediatric patient.

2. Describe the role of the professional nurse when administering medications to infants and children. Identify four safeguards to ensure accurate dosage and administration. Identify two legal and two professional implications of unsafe or inaccurate administration of medications.

3. Advocating for a child in pain is a role of the professional nurse. List three behavioral assessments that denote pain in each of the following age groups: infants, toddlers, and preschoolers; school-age children; and adolescents. Describe how you would determine which analgesic to administer if oral or intramuscular medications were ordered. List assessments or criteria that would assist you in determining the medication route.

4. Using the diagnosis, anxiety related to fear of needles and injections, initiate a care plan for a newly diagnosed eight-year-old diabetic. Describe the assessment data used to substantiate the diagnosis, define interventions to assist the pediatric client, and document outcome criteria for evaluation.

MULTIPLE CHOICE ITEMS

1. Factors affecting the potency of a drug's action(s) include:

a. Health status of the client
b. Organ maturity
c. Body surface
d. Genetic endowment
1. a, b, c
2. a, c
3. b, c, d
4. b, d
*5. All of the above

2. When calculating a drug dose for a pediatric client using the surface rule, the following information is necessary:

a. Adult dose of medication
b. A nomogram
c. Age of the child
d. Suggested dose for child's weight
*1. a, b
2. a, c
3. b, d
4. c, d

CALCULATIONS

1. A pediatric client has the following sedation ordered for an invasive procedure:

20 mg	Meperidine
10 mg	Promethazine
10 mg	Chlorpromazine

You have vials of the following:

50 mg/1 cc	Meperidine
25 mg/1 cc	Promethazine
25 mg/1 cc	Chlorpromazine

How many cc's of each medication will you prepare?

Answers:

0.4 cc's	Meperidine
0.4 cc's	Promethazine
0.4 cc's	Chlorpromazine

2. The usual dose of an antibiotic is 20 mg/kg/24 hours. The child weighs 30 kilograms. Determine the maximum individual dose if the child was to receive the medication every 8 hours.

Answer: 20 mg X 30 kg = 600 mg/24 hours
600 mg/24° + 3 doses = 200 mg/dose

TRUE AND FALSE STATEMENTS

_F_ **1.** Play therapy allays a child's fear of medication administration but is not effective with chronically ill children.

_F_ **2.** Mature renal and hepatic systems in young children assist with the effective use of medication.

_T_ **3.** The surface rule provides one of the safest and more accurate measures for determining pediatric medication doses.

_T_ **4.** The professional nurse is responsible for calculating doses to ensure accuracy of the written medication order.

51
Drug Therapy in Gerontologic Nursing

Chapter 51 describes factors that may predispose elderly clients to unfavorable drug effects. Guidelines are presented for the student to consider for the promotion of good medication habits and prevention of adverse reactions. The text helps the student to develop a holistic approach in assessing medication use among elderly clients.

Through the study of this chapter, students may develop the following concepts:

1 □ There are several factors relevant to elderly clients that predispose them to risk of medication administration errors.
2 □ Normal physiologic changes associated with the aging process may influence the body's ability to handle drugs.
3 □ Drug toxicity in elderly clients may not follow a predictable pattern.
4 □ The coordinated efforts of the nurse, physician, and pharmacist are essential to produce an optimum safe medication regimen for elderly clients.
5 □ A holistic drug history and assessment are essential for helping the elderly client and family establish an optimum medication regimen.
6 □ The role of the nurse includes client advocacy, client–family teaching, and coordination of the health team to ensure maximum safe medication use by the elderly client.

Teaching Strategies

1 □ Review classifications of drugs that may not be completely eliminated because of impaired or reduced renal and hepatic function (*e.g.*, antibiotics, sulfonamides, and aminoglycosides.)
2 □ Assign students three to five elderly clients and instruct them to interview the clients regarding number and types of medications, diagnoses (past and present), and other health-related problems. Follow this activity with a class session in which students summarize and compare their results. Students may find clients in senior housing units, senior citizens' centers, nutrition centers, proprietary homes, and health-related facilities.
3 □ Use the information obtained above to determine the cost of medications for one elderly client during a period of 1 month.
4 □ Have students take thorough medication assessments for one elderly client and then discuss the risk-to-benefit ratio for each drug they are taking.
5 □ Use anecdotes to illustrate the role of the nurse in promoting the safe effective use of medications in the following setting:

a. Housing facilities for the elderly (group classes related to common drugs prescribed, office hours).
b. Nutrition centers (classes with specific days for clients to bring in all medications for review).
c. Elderly clients of Hispanic origin living in a predominantly Spanish-speaking community (cultural factors that influence drug use).
d. Elderly clients admitted to an acute care setting. Divide the class into small groups of four to eight students to discuss and outline the specific role of the nurse in these settings.

6 □ Invite pharmacists from several settings (*e.g.*, acute care, skilled nursing facility [SNF], neighborhood drugstore, mental health facility) to present a panel discussion on their role in promoting safe effective use of medications among their elderly clients.

Evaluation Examples (Test Items)

ESSAY QUESTIONS

1. Describe why the following drugs used for elderly clients require close supervision and monitoring by the nurse:

a. Digoxin
b. Antibiotics
c. Aminoglycosides

(Note: You may consult a drug reference for data on these agents.)

2. Ms. RM is an 80-year-old widow of Italian heritage who lives with her 58-year-old daughter in a low-income residential neighborhood. Her diagnoses include stasis dermatitis, CHF, ASHD, hypothyroidism, and rheumatoid arthritis. The drugs she is taking are digoxin, Lasix, Dalmane, Darvon, KCl, $FeSO_4$, and Synthroid. Identify and describe the important factors that must be considered in planning a safe medication regimen for this client.

MULTIPLE CHOICE ITEMS

1. The following factors must be considered when assessing a client's medication regimen:

a. Renal functioning
b. Lean body weight
c. Behavioral changes
d. Mental status
e. Financial resources
1. a, b, c
2. a, c, d
3. b, d, e
*4. All of the above

2. Elderly clients are at an increased risk of drug toxicity because
a. The prescriber may be unaware of all the drugs that the client is taking
b. Presenting signs of toxicity may be viewed as normal signs of aging
c. They frequently share the medications of family or friends
d. They more often request medications to relieve minor aches and pains
1. b, c
2. b, c, d
*3. a, b, c
4. All of the above

3. When planning a teaching program for the medication regimen of an elderly client living with family, the nurse should
a. Take a thorough drug history, including use of over-the-counter drugs and home remedies
b. Advise the family to use childproof caps at all times to prevent accidental poisoning
c. Avoid talking too much about side effects because it only confuses and scares the client and family
d. Schedule medication administration times to coincide with daily routine as much as possible
1. b, c
2. a, b
*3. a, d
4. All of the above

52 Drug Therapy in Community Health Nursing

The scope of drug use in the home should include all substances having a potential pharmacologic or deleterious effect on the body. Students should be encouraged to consider a wide variety of drug sources such as air, water, and soil pollution, household plants and chemicals, food preparations, and personal care products. The use of over-the-counter products such as antacids, analgesics, and laxative products should be explored, as well as the possible use of illicit drugs. Some students may feel that taking a thorough drug history is beyond the role of the community health nurse. These students could be instructed to define the role of the professional nurse in the current health-care delivery system and to outline the functions of a responsible health-care provider in the administration and monitoring of drugs. The learning experiences included in Chapter 52 address this issue and are offered to illuminate the role of the community health nurse.

By studying this chapter, the student should develop the following concepts:

1 □ The nurse plays a specific role in teaching and assessing the client regarding drug use in the home.
2 □ Certain client variables affect self-administration and compliance to the drug therapy regimen.
3 □ A drug history should be based on a broad definition of drugs that includes household plants, chemicals, and other ingestible products.
4 □ The administration of drugs and their effects in the home setting should be monitored by the nurse.
5 □ The nurse should be familiar with techniques that enhance both compliance and the proper storage of drugs.

Teaching Strategies

As early as possible in the curriculum, students should be introduced to the idea that safe drug use involves the shared responsibility of client, nurse, physician, pharmacist, and researcher. Students should be reintroduced to this concept as they acquire a broader knowledge of pharmacology and a more in-depth understanding of the pharmaceutic effects of many substances. It is important for them to review their own beliefs about drugs, about how they should be taken—from a consumer's perspective—and administered—from a nurse's perspective. Equally important is the value they place on health-care maintenance—specifically, through the use of drugs. Their approach to clients in the home and in community-based practice requires a broad definition of drugs, a basic appreciation of motivational theory, and a solid grasp of their own health-care values. It is suggested that all students take a home drug history of a client or family, preferably toward the end of their studies, to allow them to apply and integrate previous knowledge about health behaviors and family and professional roles, as well as of pharmacology. Some of the following strategies may be used to enhance the student's appreciation of the dynamic interrelationship between client and family variables, community perspectives on drugs, and current drug knowledge:

1 □ Help students to apply Rosenstock's health belief model regarding clients' perceived susceptibility to disease and the seriousness of the disease to drug use and self-care in the home. The students may assess their own drug-taking behavior as it relates to these factors.
2 □ Divide the class into pairs and have them interview a pharmacist and community health nurse. Then have them compare their impressions regarding the roles of each, emphasizing the teaching role of the health-care provider.
3 □ Use role play with a client drug history interview to depict a person who is somewhat forgetful and who keeps medications in various places throughout the home. Have other faculty members or experienced students participate.
4 □ Ask students to list the community resources that aid the following at-risk populations to take drugs correctly: elderly, disabled, low economic status, and handicapped.

Evaluation Examples (Test Items)

ESSAY QUESTIONS

1. Outline an approach to taking a drug history in the home of a chronically ill client whose spouse sometimes administers the multiple drugs prescribed.

2. List and discuss the ways of evaluating a client's compliance with a drug regimen when fear of side effects is suspected.

SHORT ANSWER QUESTIONS

1. List five client variables that reflect the client's knowledge of the drugs being taken. (Administration, regimen, action, effects, side effects, contraindications)

2. Name four ways in which a prescription label is identified. (Client's name and address, physician's name, pharmacy's name, prescription number)

MULTIPLE CHOICE ITEMS

1. Which of the following factors does *not* affect drug use in the home?

1. Attitudes about self-care
2. Previous experience with drugs
3. Recent hospitalization
4. Health status

*5. None of the above

2. The nurse could prevent drug misuse in the home by which of the following measures?

*1. Establish a check-and-balance system (*e.g.*, family or neighbor)

2. Give own home phone number for emergency care
3. Call daily to remind client to take medication
4. Alert the hospital emergency room for possible adverse response

3. When taking a drug history, the nurse must be aware of which of the following important factors?

a. Previous drug reactions, over-the-counter drugs, daily habits, dietary patterns
b. Names of all doctors, plants in the home, and household chemicals used
c. Diagnoses, physical and sensory impairments, and allergies

1. a, b
2. b, c
3. a, c

*4. All of the above

4. When a client is experiencing difficulty in remembering to take medications, which of the following methods would be most appropriate for the community health nurse to use?

a. Seeking a family member or significant other to be responsible for dispensing all his medications
b. Making weekly visits to set up all the client's medications for the week in an egg carton
c. Asking the prescriber to cut down on the client's medications and give only essential medications as few times a day as possible
d. Explaining why each medication must be taken and then phoning daily until the client adapts to the routine

*1. a, b

2. a, c
3. b, d
4. None of the above

53 Drug Therapy for Pain Relief

Chapter 53 considers the nursing management of analgesia in three common clinical situations: acute short-term pain, chronic pain, and pain in the terminally ill. Common causes for failure to achieve effective pain relief are also discussed.

Through the study of this chapter, students may develop the following concepts:

1 □ Because pain is in large part a subjective experience, nurses must give credence to clients' subjective descriptions of their pain.
2 □ Correction of the cause of pain is preferable to palliative analgesia.
3 □ Although pain threshold is similar for most people, pain perception varies greatly from person to person and from time to time in the same person.
4 □ Pain perception is influenced by multiple factors, including underlying pathology, stress responses, and conditioning in previous pain experiences.
5 □ Use of analgesics is a conditioned response, learned through positive reinforcement when a pain stimulus is allowed to reach a discomforting level and is subsequently alleviated by medication.
6 □ Repeated stimulation of a pain pathway facilitates transmission of nerve impulses along that pathway; this constitutes a physiologic habit of pain.
7 □ Response to stress may increase or decrease perception of pain.
8 □ Medication ordered PRN may be administered prophylactically when client need is predictable.
9 □ Optimal analgesia requires planning for medication at optimal times.
10 □ The overall amount of analgesic drugs required for alleviation of pain is least when pain is not allowed to reach discomforting levels.
11 □ Psychologic dependence on drugs is more difficult to treat than is physical dependence.
12 □ Personal attitudes of nurses toward the use of analgesics influence their management of analgesic medication unless they are consciously aware of their biases and take measures to compensate for them.
13 □ Placebos induce real physical changes in the body that underly their efficacy.

Teaching Strategies

1 □ A study of this unit could be integrated within a unit on pain that incorporates both pharmacologic and nonpharmacologic nursing approaches to the alleviation of pain. Emphasis should be placed on combining these two types of care, rather than dichotomizing and using either drugs and comfort measures separately.
2 □ Topics for classroom discussion could include the following:

- **a.** Personal attitudes toward the use of analgesic drugs, their influence on nursing judgments, and measures for minimizing bias as a factor in the planning of nursing care of clients in pain. Students are more willing to acknowledge bias if instructors share their own and the measures they employ to minimize their influence on nursing care. Discussion is facilitated if all participants attempt to clarify their attitudes prior to class time (a written assignment may help to ensure this; the written material need not be handed in).
- **b.** Client situations drawn from students' or instructors' clinical experience.
- **c.** Personal pain experiences illustrative of the factors influencing pain perception.

Evaluation Examples (Test Items)

MULTIPLE CHOICE ITEMS

1. Drugs used to relieve pain include
   a. Antacids
   b. Muscle relaxants
   c. Prostaglandin antagonists
   d. Opiates
   1. a, b, c
   2. a, b, d
   3. a, c, d
   4. b, c, d
   *5. All of the above

2. Pain threshold
   *1. Is the same for most people
   2. Varies from person to person
   3. Varies from time to time in the same person
   4. Both 2 and 3 above

3. Pain perception
   1. Is the same for most people

2. Varies from person to person
3. Varies from time to time in the same person
*4. Both 2 and 3 above

4. Pain perception is usually greatest
1. In the early morning hours, after awakening
*2. In the evening and night hours
3. When the client is subject to various stimuli, whether pleasant or unpleasant
4. None of the above; pain perception tends to be constant

5. When a client requires analgesic drugs in greater amounts than usually required by clients with similar conditions, the nurse should
1. Accept the client's assessment of need and request an order for a larger dose or stronger form of analgesic
*2. Assess the client carefully for complications that may underly the increase in perceived pain
3. Discuss the risks of dependence on analgesic drugs with the client
4. Administer a placebo to determine whether the client has developed psychologic dependence on the drug

6. Overt responses to pain include
a. An elevation of blood pressure
b. A decrease in blood pressure
c. An increase in activity levels
d. A decrease in activity levels
1. a, b
2. a, c
3. b, c
4. b, d
*5. All of the above

7. Chronic pain is best controlled by
1. Using the least amount of the least potent analgesic tolerable
2. Administering pain medication intermittently, as required by pain level
3. Enlisting the client's cooperation in keeping drug use to a minimum
*4. Administering initial doses greater than those expected to alleviate the symptoms, subsequently lowering doses to the minimum amount required for pain control.

SITUATION-BASED MULTIPLE CHOICE ITEMS

Situation: Ms. CM, age 48 years, had a cholecystectomy yesterday. She has T-tube drainage of the common bile duct and a drain in the wound. The intravenous infusion is to be discontinued when a full liquid diet can be taken, but as yet she is tolerating only clear fluids. She is to get out of bed for the first time this morning. During breakfast, CM complains of "quite a bad pain" in the operative area, which has been increasing steadily for the last half hour.

1. To clarify the nature of her pain further, you should
1. Check the site of the intravenous infusion for extravasation
2. Scrutinize CM's sclerae for jaundice
3. Check the wound for dehiscence
*4. Check the T tube for patency

2. CM's pain is not relieved by repositioning. She has not had any pain medication since 10 PM the previous night. Your best action would be to
1. Ambulate CM and administer the analgesic drug immediately after she returns to bed
*2. Administer the opioid analgesic and allow CM to rest undisturbed until the pain subsides
3. Administer the opioid analgesic and obtain help to ambulate CM while the drug is at peak action
4. Administer the opioid analgesic and wait until afternoon to ambulate CM

3. CM tells you that she slept very poorly the previous night because of persistent incisional discomfort. You would advise her, should the pain recur, to
1. Request a sleeping pill from the night nurse
*2. Request pain medication at bedtime if she has any discomfort
3. Request pain medication whenever the pain becomes severe
4. Take a dose of aspirin from the supply in her purse if she has discomfort at bedtime

4. CM expresses reluctance to use "dope" unless she "really needs it." You should tell her that
a. Pain increases the risk of postoperative complications, including infection
b. Pain delays healing
c. If drug dependence develops, it will be relatively easy to overcome because the drugs were used medicinally instead of for their psychotropic effect
*1. a, b
2. a, c
3. b, c
4. All of the above

5. The postoperative complications that are more likely to develop in those whose pain is not well controlled include
a. Hypotensive shock
b. Infection
c. Dehiscence
d. Abnormal clotting (thrombophlebitis)
1. a, d
2. b, c
3. b only
4. a, c, d
*5. All of the above

6. The physiologic mechanisms by which pain influences the risk of postoperative complications include the following body responses to stress:
a. Reflex vasodilation
b. Increased secretion of epinephrine
c. Increased secretion of glucocorticoids
d. Increased secretion of growth hormone
*1. a, b, c
2. a, b, d

3. a, c, d
4. b, c, d

7. On the third morning after surgery, CM requests "her pain shot." She had required only one injection for pain the previous day, after ambulating in the late afternoon. She describes her pain as "feeling awful all over." Your best response is to

1. Administer the opioid analgesic promptly
2. Avoid giving the opioid by using physical comfort measures to alleviate CM's discomfort

*3. Request an order for a nonnarcotic analgesic, such as aspirin
4. Teach CM relaxation and self-hypnosis techniques to alleviate her discomfort

54 Self-Medication with Over-the-Counter Drugs

Legislative Controls
Characteristics of Nonprescription Drugs
Nursing Management
Nursing Implications
Nursing Process

Chapter 54 introduces the student to drugs that are sold without prescription and that are used by lay people for self-medication. Legal regulations on the manufacturing, labeling, and advertising of these products are described; guidelines are presented for optimal use of these substances. The chapter concludes with a discussion of nursing management.

Through the study of this chapter, the student may develop the following concepts:

1 □ Legal regulations controlling the production and marketing of over-the-counter drugs are designed to ensure minimal safety and efficacy of drug products offered for sale without medical supervision.
2 □ A limited number of chemical agents are approved for use in over-the-counter preparations; drug firms tend to exploit these drugs fully by incorporating them into many preparations and using them for different therapeutic effects.
3 □ Doses recommended for over-the-counter drugs are usually in the low therapeutic range.
4 □ In attempts to enhance effectiveness and reduce side effects, manufacturers of over-the-counter drugs often combine several drugs agents in each preparation.
5 □ The dosage of drugs in multiple drug combinations with fixed dosages cannot be adjusted to meet individual needs of clients.
6 □ The use of inappropriate multiple drug combinations leads to excessive medication.
7 □ Warning statements on the labels of over-the-counter preparations are required by law for minimal safety and should be carefully heeded.
8 □ Terminology on drug labels may be difficult to interpret (for both lay and professional people).
9 □ Although controlled to a degree by legal regulations, advertising and labeling are designed to promote the use of over-the-counter drugs.
10 □ Over-the-counter preparations are helpful in alleviating minor short-term illnesses and the symptoms of stable chronic illness.
11 □ When symptoms for which over-the-counter drugs are used become more severe, or when they persist beyond the usual time for recovery, definitive diagnosis by health professionals should be sought.
12 □ Prolonged use or excessive dosage of over-the-counter preparations can lead to serious illnesses.

Teaching Strategies

The study of nonprescription drugs is most pertinent to community nursing, because members of this nursing specialty are usually more involved in counseling clients about self-care practices than are nurses in other specialties. The study of this chapter, along with Chapter 52, would be appropriate within the context of a course on community nursing.

Some of the learning and enrichment experiences direct students to explore the shelves of local drugstores to become familiar with the drug preparations offered for sale. Prior arrangements for these activities should be made with the proprietors and pharmacists of local establishments. A schedule may be needed to prevent flooding of a store with large numbers of students. Students should be cautioned to avoid requests for assistance from, or prolonged discussions with, busy personnel in the stores. It may be appropriate to schedule these experiences as part of the laboratory experience and to develop formal guidelines for the student experience.

Data gathered by students during the field assignments provide a basis for classroom discussion. Personal experience of faculty and students, as well as client situations involving over-the-counter drugs, can further enrich the discussions.

Evaluation Examples (Test Items)

ESSAY QUESTIONS

1. Briefly describe the federal laws regulating the manufacturing and sale of nonprescription drugs in the United States.

2. What recommendations would you make to a client who expresses concern about the long-standing use of heavy doses of proprietary antacid preparations by her husband?

3. Briefly discuss the advantages and disadvantages of using nonprescription medications for self-medication. Identify guidelines for optimal use of these preparations.

MULTIPLE CHOICE ITEMS

1. The legislation that defined legend (prescription) and over-the-counter (nonprescription) drugs was
1. The Food, Drug, and Cosmetic Act of 1906
2. The Food, Drug, and Cosmetic Act of 1938
*3. The Durham-Humphrey Amendment of 1952
4. The Controlled Substance Act of 1970

2. The federal agency that enforces the regulations pertaining to over-the-counter drugs is
1. The Federal Narcotic Control Commission
2. The Treasury Department
3. The Controlled Substance Commission
*4. The Food and Drug Administration

3. Characteristics of over-the-counter drugs include
a. Selection of drug ingredients from a list that includes most of the therapeutic agents available for prescription
b. Use of multiple substances combined in a single preparation
c. Use of agents for physiologic effects normally considered in medical practice to be side effects of the drug
1. a, b
*2. b, c
3. a, c
4. All of the above
5. None of the above

4. Most over-the-counter cold and sinus preparations contain a combination of
1. Sedatives, laxatives, and aspirin
2. Antihistamines, scopolamine, and stimulants
3. Expectorants, decongestants, and hypnotics
*4. Antihistamines, sympathomimetics, and aspirin

SITUATION-BASED MULTIPLE CHOICE ITEMS

Situation: Your neighbor, Ms. MT, expresses concern about her husband's (FT's) use of "patent medicines," especially aspirin and antacids. She asks you if "all that medicine" is "good for anyone."

1. You should first determine
a. What the symptoms are for which the drugs are taken
b. What dosage of the drugs her husband is taking
c. How long he has been taking the drugs
d. What brand-name drugs he is taking
*1. a, b, c
2. a, b, d
3. a, c, d
4. b, c, d
5. All of the above

2. You are told that FT began to take large doses of aspirin several weeks ago on the advice of his physician to relieve joint pains attributed to osteoarthritis. The aspirin gave him an "upset stomach" that was relieved by antacids. You might appropriately recommend that FT
1. Stop taking all medication for at least 2 weeks, and then reevaluate his condition
2. Substitute acetaminophen for the aspirin and see if he could reduce the dosage of antacids
*3. Consult the physician to see if a different antirheumatic with less stomach irritation would be effective
4. Substitute an enteric-coated aspirin preparation for the plain aspirin he has been taking

3. FT has also experienced a tendency toward constipation since taking antacids. You could tell his wife that
*1. Antacids can cause either constipation or diarrhea, depending on their active ingredients
2. FT should stop taking the antacids immediately to prevent a serious intestinal obstruction
3. The change in bowel habits is probably unrelated to the antacids
4. The change in bowel status should be immediately investigated by a gastroenterologist

4. MT asks you, with concern, whether her husband will now have to take expensive prescription drugs to control his arthritis. You could tell her that
a. Prescription drugs are usually necessary for the control of osteoarthritis
b. There are several over-the-counter antirheumatic drugs on the market that may be used to control osteoarthritis
c. Over-the-counter drugs are sometimes recommended for control of a long-term condition
d. Drug therapy for long-term conditions should be supervised by health-care professionals
1. a, b, c
2. a, b, d
3. a, c, d
*4. b, c, d
5. All of the above